DRUGS AND THEIR USAGE

BY

Dr. Will Grimley

Dr. Randy Lynn   Dr. Beth Myhre Blevins   Dr. Beth Robinson

Christian Veterinary Mission

Current Book Information at:
www.cvm.org

FIRST EDITION

This is a first edition of the Drugs and Their Usage book. We think it will meet a need that hasn't been addressed before in the developing world. The information regarding drugs is current and accurate, additionally, many practical aspects of drug use have been included. We hope it meets your expectations as well. If you have suggestions or questions concerning contents of this book, please address them to CVM, Seattle using the address given on the previous page.

Disclaimer:

This book was prepared according to the current veterinary medical literature available. It is prepared as a service to the animal producers and veterinary practitioners laboring in the veterinary mission field. The editors, authors, co-authors, and contributors to this volume, as well as Christian Veterinary Mission and World Concern assume no responsibility for and make no warranty with respect to the results that may be obtained from the uses, procedures, withdrawal periods, or dosages listed, and do not necessarily endorse such uses, procedures, withdrawal periods or dosages. Furthermore, the editors, authors, co-authors, and contributors to this volume, as well as Christian Veterinary Mission and World Concern shall not be liable to anyone whatsoever for any damage resulting from reliance on any information contained herein, whether with respect to drug identification, uses, procedures, dosages, or equivalencies, or by reason of miss-statement or error, negligent or otherwise, contained in this work.

The drugs, doses, indications, and withdrawal periods detailed in this book do not and cannot comply with the veterinary drug laws of every sovereign country. Before using any animal drugs the reader must become thoroughly familiar with the local laws and regulations that apply to drug use in animals and practice strict adherence to those laws. Similarly, this book is not intended to substitute for the complete prescribing information prepared by each manufacturer for each drug. The package insert and directions for use of every drug product should be read, understood and followed before any drug is prescribed or administered.

Raising Healthy Animals Series

Every year, thousands of people around the world struggle to survive because they don't have the right knowledge, skills and resources to care for their animals. Christian Veterinary Mission (CVM) sends veterinary professionals to live and work alongside many of these people to encourage them and provide them with not only much needed veterinary expertise, but also the hope that is only found in Christ. CVM veterinarians build lasting relationships with individuals and communities, helping them be transformed through Christ's love.

CVM, in its effort to be meaningfully involved in work in the developing world, quickly found there was little appropriate educational material available. CVM set about developing basic resource materials in animal husbandry for farmers and agricultural workers. Apparently, they met a real need, as these books have been accepted throughout the developing nations of the world.

The series of books published by Christian Veterinary Mission includes the following in order of publication:

Raising Healthy Pigs *	Drugs and Their Usage
Raising Healthy Rabbits *	Where There Is No Animal Doctor
Raising Healthy Fish	Raising Healthy Horses
Raising Healthy Cattle	Zoonoses: Animal Diseases That Affect Humans
Raising Healthy Poultry *+	Raising Healthy Honey Bees
Raising Healthy Goats *	Slaughter and Preservation of Meat
Raising Healthy Sheep	Disease and Parasite Prevention in Farm Animals

[Also available in: * Spanish + French].

CVM fieldworkers have also developed specific training materials for the countries in which they work.

All of these books have been put together by Christian men and women; in a labor of love and service, for people in need throughout the world. It demonstrates dedication to their profession, service to humanity and a witness to their faith. We hope that they are a help to you in developing an appropriate livestock program to meet your needs. We pray God's blessing on their use.

Leroy Dorminy
CVM Founder

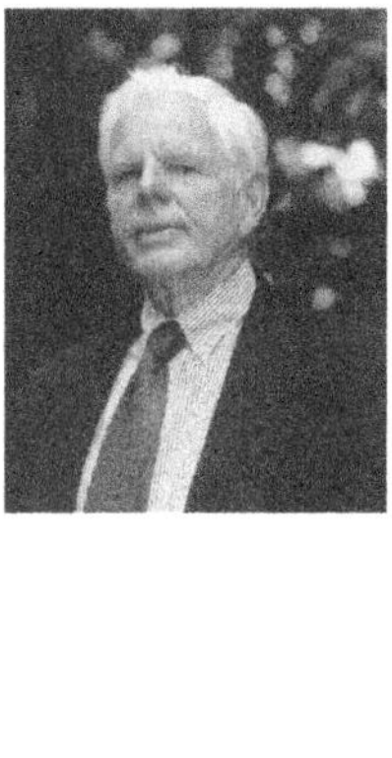

TABLE OF CONTENTS

SECTION I -- Introduction

SECTION II -- Animal Restraint

SECTION III -- Determining Drug Dosages

SECTION VII -- Drug Formulary

SECTION VIII -- Vaccines

SECTION IX -- Control of Ectoparasites

SECTION 1

INTRODUCTION

INTRODUCTION

WHO MIGHT USE THIS BOOK

Making the correct diagnosis is the most important part of treating an animal or flock. This task is often complicated and difficult and at times impossible. This book is designed to aid the veterinarian and the veterinary technician in making knowledgeable and well thought out decisions in the treatment of animals presented. There is no substitute for training in the fields of nutrition, animal care and veterinary medicine, yet the veterinarian and veterinary technician should be willing to use reference materials for help in diagnosis and treatment.

Most veterinarians or veterinary technicians cannot remember each and every detail about every medication that is available. Everyone needs a reference book to look up important information. We designed this reference book so that it could be carried into the field. The format and vocabulary are simple, although we expect improvements to be made in future editions.

Much general information has been included because of its importance in the evaluation of the animal and in the proper use of medicines. These include such items as restraint techniques, history taking, physical examination technique, methods of determining an animal's weight, and locations to give injectable drugs.

HOW TO USE THIS BOOK

First, the veterinary technician should read the entire **Table of Contents** to become familiar with the topics covered. When information is needed in the future, the technician will know if that particular topic is contained within the book.

Second, read the **glossary** located near the end of the book. This will provide a good start for learning veterinary terms used in this book and elsewhere.

Third, read the sections of interest. Look up in the **glossary** any veterinary terms which are not known. Refer to an English dictionary for the meanings of other words in the text.

The **index** should be used to find specific drugs or chemicals by their generic names. General information can be located through the **index** too.

This is not a holy book so write in it -- make notes, underline important points, add comments given by veterinarians, blot out mistakes (we tried hard not to make any!) and include items left out but which are important.

REMEMBER -- to find things quickly look in the **Table of Contents** or **index**.

WHAT IS A MEDICINE OR DRUG?

A medicine is a chemical which performs a specific job in the body. These chemicals can be man-made or harvested from plants, animals, insects or microorganisms.

Drugs are usually grouped according to their use. Even though a drug has a specific job, it can also have other effects in the body called side effects. Sometimes the side effects are helpful, but most of the time they create problems.

Specific medicines have been developed to help cure specific diseases. There is no single medicine that cures all diseases. Antibiotics are an example. There are many, many bacteria that infect animals and each antibiotic kills only certain bacteria. Therefore selecting the correct antibiotic for a specific type of bacterial infection is of great importance. The veterinary technician should know both the correct time to use a drug as well as when not to use one. Should there be any question about this, then it would be better not to use the drug!

Medicines alone cannot cure a health problem, but must work along with the body to succeed. Therefore, it is very important that the body get proper care -- good food, fresh water, adequate rest, and comfortable surroundings -- as well as the proper medicine.

The proverb which states -- "An ounce of prevention is worth a pound of cure." -- rings true in the field of animal health. Most animals or birds which are adequately fed, offered clean water, and put under as little stress as possible will naturally fight disease much more effectively compared to those who are continually struggling to find food, unspoiled water, rest, and relief from insects.

Take care of your animal and he will take care of himself and you.

WHAT IS DISEASE ?

The dictionary says disease is a deviation of the body from its normal or healthy state. There are hundreds of deviations (diseases) which the body can undergo. Some of these diseases are worse than others. Some diseases are curable, others lead to a quick death, and still others take years to develop to the stage where they are causing a problem.

One set of symptoms in an animal can be caused by many different disease conditions. The broad categories of causes of disease are:

Anomalies. An example is an umbilical hernia.

Degenerative disorders. An example is cataracts of an old dog.

Infectious. An example is tetanus in a horse.

Metabolic. An example is milk fever in a cow.

Nutritional. An example is rickets (Vitamin D deficiency).

Cancer. An example would be cancer eye in cattle.

When a veterinarian or veterinary technician is presented with a sick animal, he should think of all the possible causes. Using the above list of categories to list the causes, taking a thorough history about the animal, performing a complete physical exam, and knowing the most common local diseases will lead to a diagnosis. One should note that some diseases must be diagnosed with laboratory testing or necropsy.

WHAT HAPPENS TO A DRUG WHEN IT IS GIVEN TO AN ANIMAL OR BIRD?

The goal of drug therapy is to maintain a level of drug at the site of the disease which will be effective in treating the disease. This involves many variables including dose, how often the drug is given, the method it is given, the animal's overall health, and how quickly the drug is eliminated from the body.

After a drug is given to an animal it must cross over many barriers to reach the site of action. The medicine is first taken up by the blood vessels which are closest to where the medicine is given. For example, if medicine is given by mouth then it enters the blood after passing through the intestinal wall. If medicine is given by injection, then it enters the blood vessels in the muscle or beneath the skin. Once in the blood the drug is carried throughout the body, including to the part that is diseased. When the drug in the blood reaches a high level, it then crosses over the vessel wall into the tissues of the animal's body and does its work.

Factors which affect a drug's movement **into** and **around** the body:

1. How well it dissolves in lipids (fats)
2. The electrical charge on the drug (acid or base)
3. The size and shape of the chemicals which make up the drug
4. The degree of the animal's illness. This would include body temperature, nutritional status, energy level, and protein level in the blood.
5. Competition in the blood and body tissues by toxins or other drugs
6. How much of the drug is in the body already
7. The degree of blood flow to the area of the body that is diseased. This is influenced by hydration, edema, shock, and the anatomy of that area.
8. How well the drug dissolves in water
9. Diarrhea or constipation if the drug is taken orally
10. A drug's interaction with another substance. Antacids, mineral oil, food, milk and other drugs might interact with a medicine given orally.
11. Normal variation which exists from animal to animal even of the same species
12. How well the animal's kidneys and liver are working

To be removed from the body most drugs must be changed chemically. The liver is the most important organ with this task. Some drugs are put into the bile by the liver. They then pass out of the body through the intestinal tract and into the feces. More often, drugs are changed chemically and are eliminated through the kidneys into the urine. This process begins when the drug first enters the bloodstream and continues until it is all removed.

Residues of drugs in the body tissues, **especially the meat and milk**, can pose human health problems. These problems usually involve allergic reactions in people who consume meat or milk which contain tiny amounts of medicines from an animal's treatment. Strictly following the label directions should prevent this type of problem.

WITHDRAWAL TIMES MUST BE OBEYED SO THAT THESE HEALTH PROBLEMS WILL NOT OCCUR IN PEOPLE BECAUSE OF DRUG RESIDUES.

SECTION 2

ANIMAL RESTRAINT

ANIMAL RESTRAINT

This chapter has been taken from "Restraint of Animals"
by Dr. John R. Leahy.

BASIC ROPE WORK

Before attempting to restrain animals one must be familiar with the handling of rope and be able to tie quickly the commonly used knots. In the descriptions of the knots and restraints which follow, reference will be made to the various parts of a rope. These are the "end", which is the short piece, and the "standing part", which is the longer piece. When a rope is doubled, a "bight" is formed. A closed bight or complete circle is a "loop".

The simplest knot, and one which is the basis for many others, is the overhand knot. (fig. 2.1) It may be tied in a single rope or on a bight, (fig. 2.2) as illustrated.

Parts of the Rope

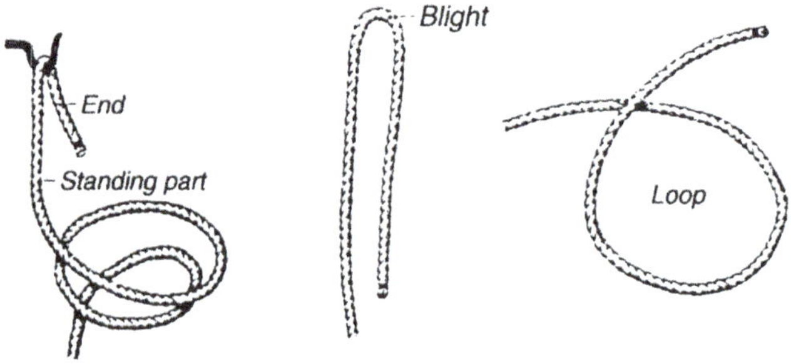

Overhand Knot

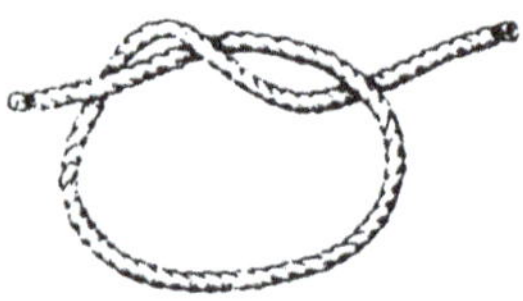

fig. 2.1

Overhand Knot Doubled

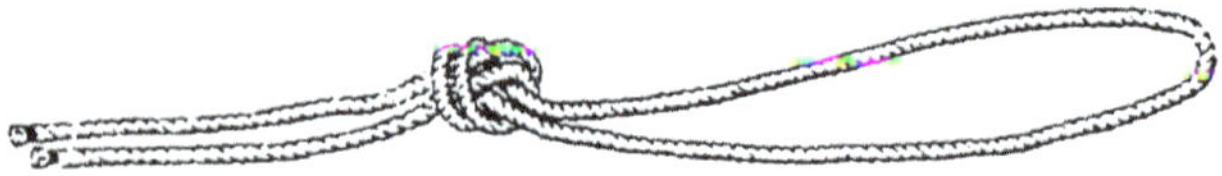

fig. 2.2

Knots for Joining Two Pieces of Rope

Cross the end of the left rope over and around the end of the right rope to make an overhand knot. (figs. 2.3 & 2.4)

Cross the new right end over and then around the new left, making a second overhand knot, pull tight. (figs. 2.5, 2.6 & 2.7)

Square Knot

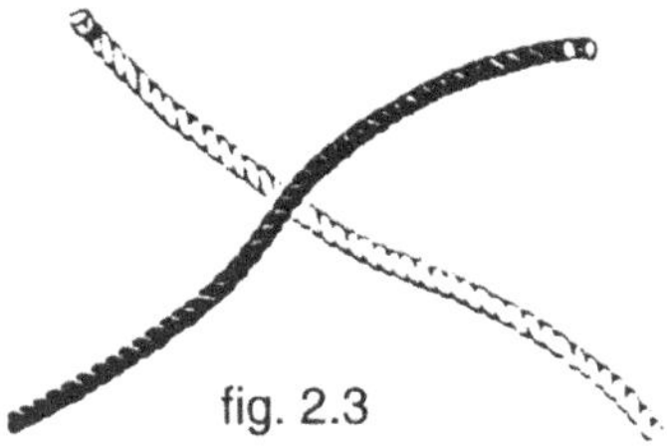

fig. 2.3

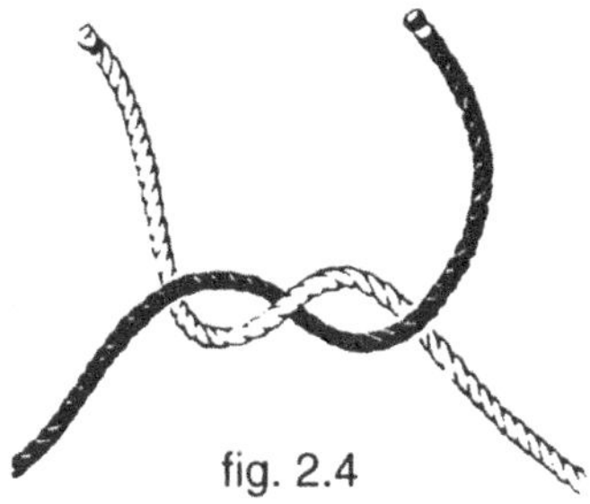

fig. 2.4

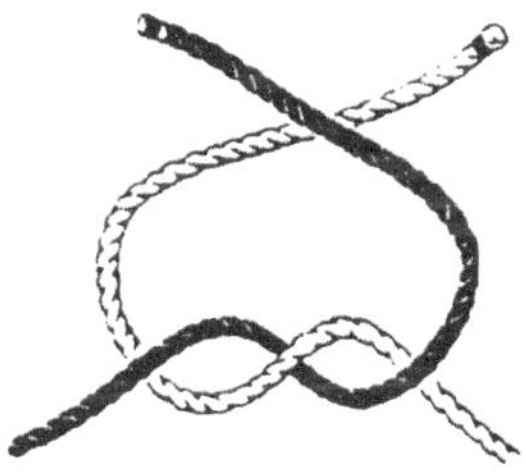

fig. 2.5

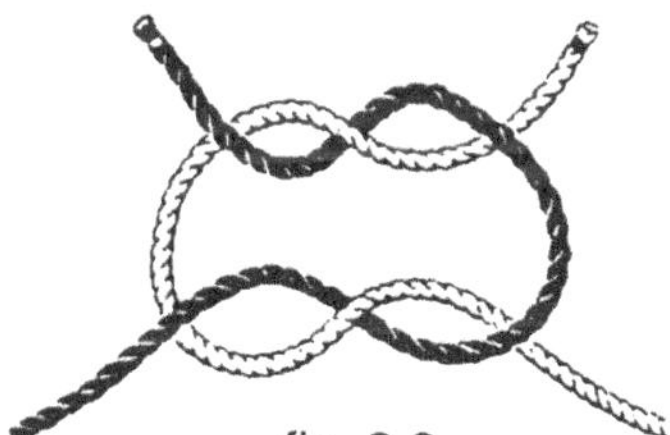

fig. 2.6

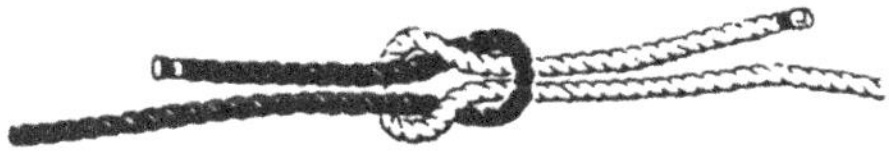

fig. 2.7

Temporary Fastenings

Bowline

The bowline is one of the most useful of all knots. It will never slip, and therefore, can be used to make a loop or noose which will not "draw down" or tighten.

- Make a loop in the standing part. (fig. 2.8)
- Pass the end through the loop and over the standing part.
- Reach under the standing part, grasp the end, bring it under the standing part and then through the loop, as indicated by the arrows. (figs. 2.9 & 2.10)
- To tighten the knot pull both the standing part and the end. (fig. 2.11)

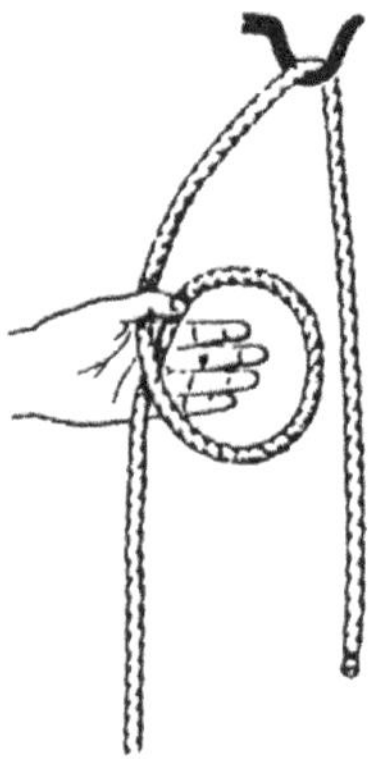

fig. 2.8

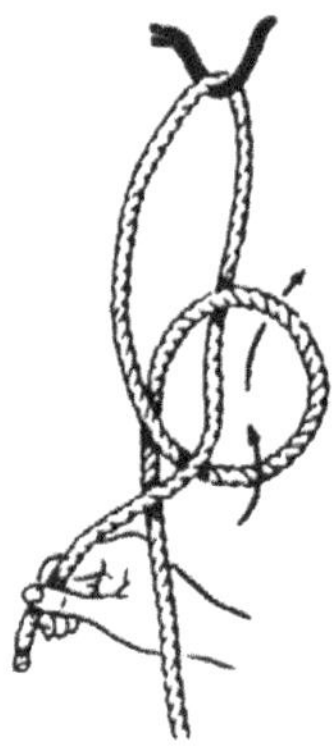

fig. 2.9

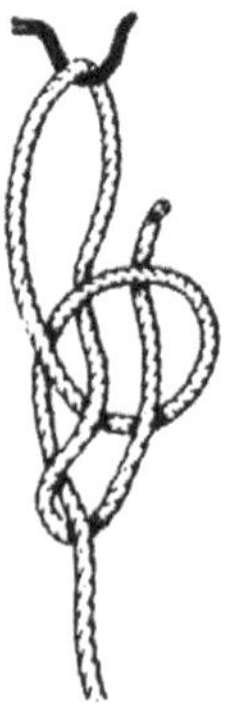

fig. 2.10

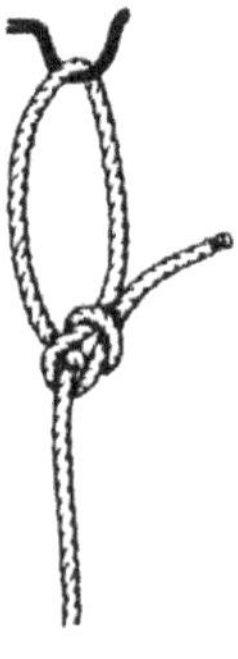

fig. 2.11

This knot may be used to tie a halter rope to a post, hook or ring, but it is inconvenient as it is not easy to untie.

- Pass the rope over or through the object to which it is to be fastened in such a way that the end will be on the right. (fig. 2.12)
- Rest the standing part on the left hand. Make a loop in the end and place it over the standing part. (fig. 2.13)
- With the right hand pass the end behind the standing part and upward through the loop. Pull the end tight. (figs. 2.14 & 2.15)
- Hold the standing part with one hand, and with the other push the knot up against the hook. (fig. 2.16)

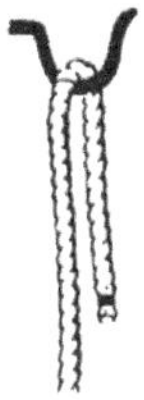

fig. 2.12

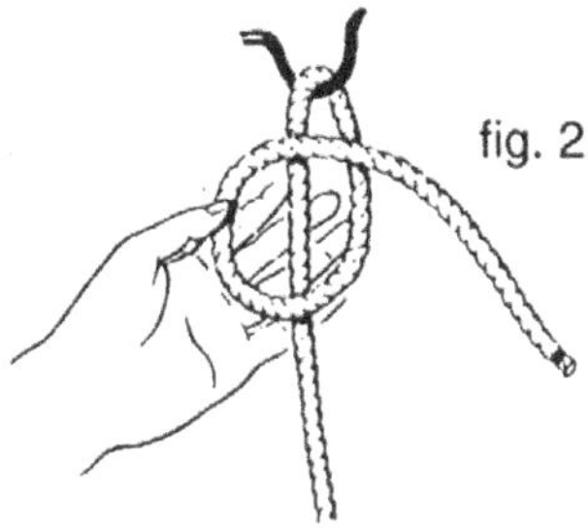

fig. 2.13

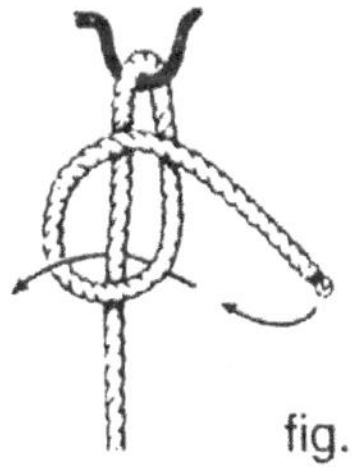

fig. 2.14

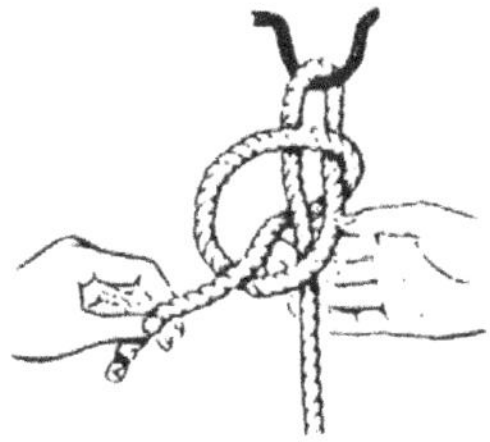

fig. 2.15

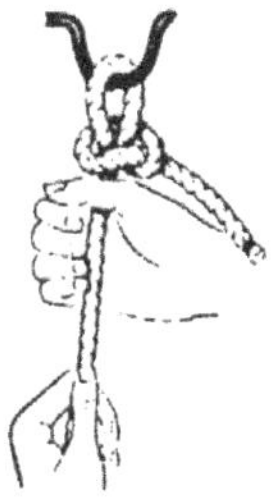

fig. 2.16

HORSE RESTRAINT

Horses, due to their size, strength and speed, are potentially dangerous animals. They are able to inflict fatal injuries easily, and they cannot be controlled by force alone. They are not necessarily hard to handle, however, if the peculiarities of their nature are understood and the many differences between individuals, noticed and respected.

Horses are nervous and suspicious themselves and are quick to detect nervousness or lack of authority in anyone else. They are apt to misinterpret any abrupt actions and to become excited. On the other hand, a direct and confident approach tends to calm them. They appreciate kindness and a tempting piece of sugar or some tasty oats will move a horse quicker than a threat, and a little scratching on the ears and even-voiced discussion will convince him quicker than shouts.

Whenever possible, one should approach a horse on his near (left) side as he is used to that. Once he is in hand, the restraint to be used should be applied confidently and quickly. In most cases it helps if the handler reasons with the horse and carries on a conversation with him as he works.

The horse can be restrained in a number of ways which vary in simplicity from twitches and hobbles to casting harnesses. Twitches distract a horse's attention; hobbles fetter his legs so that his movement is limited. Casting harnesses throw him down and confine him completely.

The restraint used should be selected to suit the horse's temperament whenever possible and, in general, no more restraint should be used than is necessary. Other things to consider in choosing a particular restraint are the horse's age and size, the location on his body of the work to be done, the length of time that the operation will take, and the amount of pain that may be inflicted. Painful operations, whether they be short or long in duration, may require sedatives as well as restraint.

In some cases, there are several different restraint techniques described which will accomplish the same purpose. Because a horse may become familiar enough with one method to be able to resist it, it is well to know as many of these as possible.

Twitches

The twitch is one of the oldest, simplest and most commonly used methods of restraint. Although there are many types of twitches, the principle which makes them effective is the same; pressure is applied to the sensory nerves of the lips and the pain produced diverts the horse's attention while less painful work is being done elsewhere on his body. Much work can be done on some horses with no restraint other than a twitch; other horses may become more intractable when a twitch is applied.

When applied too tightly or too long, twitches may become brutal instruments as they may break the skin or otherwise injure the horse's lips. They ought never to be used on horses' ears as they may permanently damage the nerves to the ear muscles.

For horses that strike, pick ax handles are good to provide more length.

One can tap on a twitch with another stick for irregular pain pulses to demand the horse's attention.

Ring Twitch

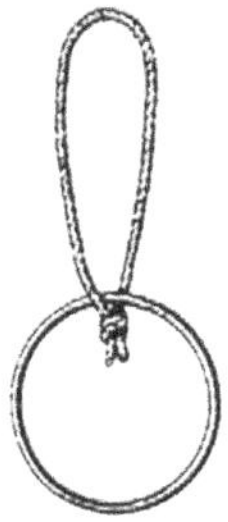

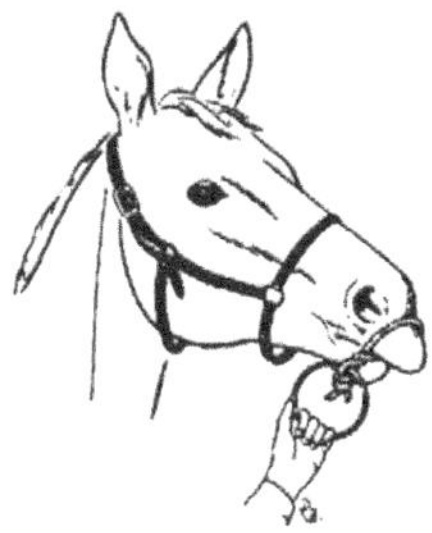

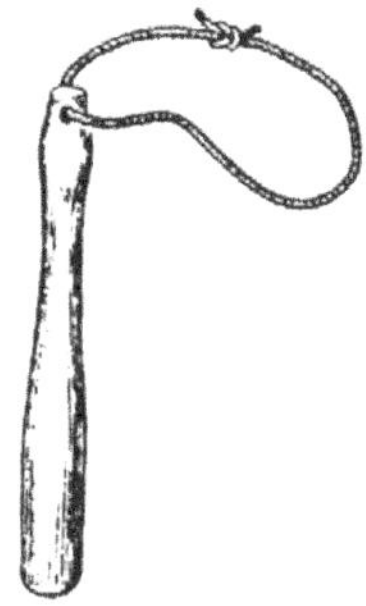

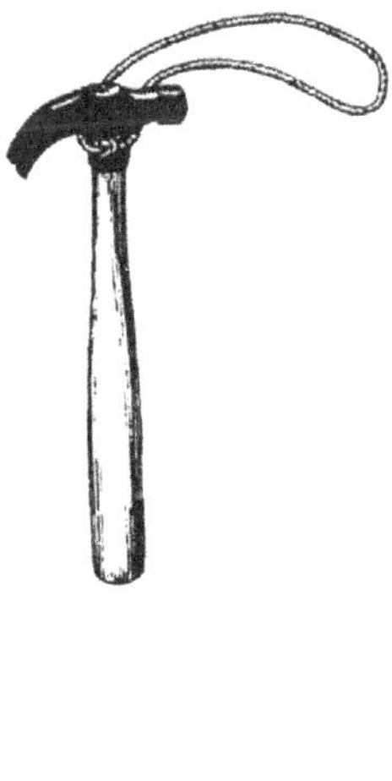

Commercial Twitch

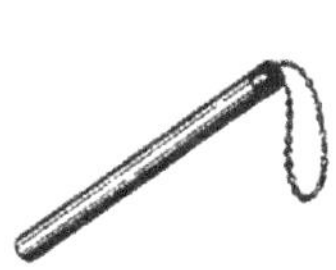

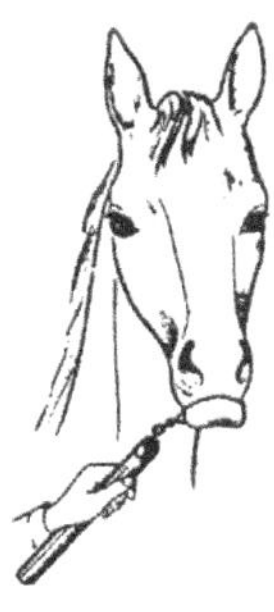

Rope Loop with a Stick Twitch

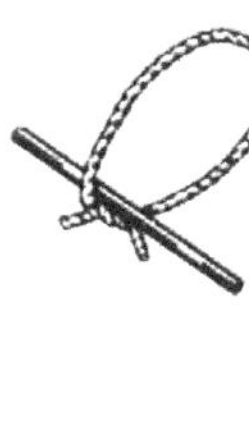

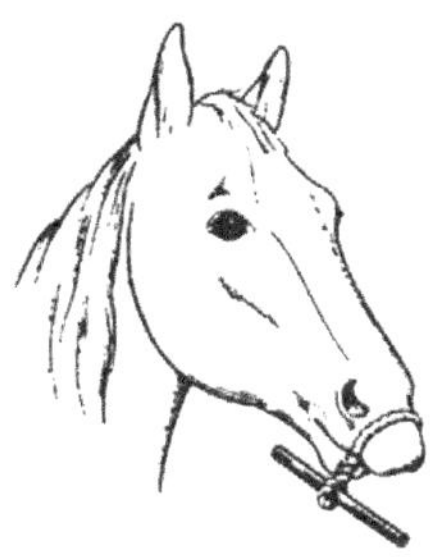

Hobbles

A hobble is a band of woven rope or leather which is placed around an animal's leg to fetter it. It may have a rope attached to it or metal rings through which a rope passes. It is better to place a hobble rather than a rope around a limb, for a rope working over the surface of the skin may injure it. Also, in moving around, a horse cannot free his leg from a hobble as easily as he could from a rope.

Pastern Hobble

This is a heavy leather strap which is adjustable at the buckle. It has a large "D" - shaped ring sewn into it.

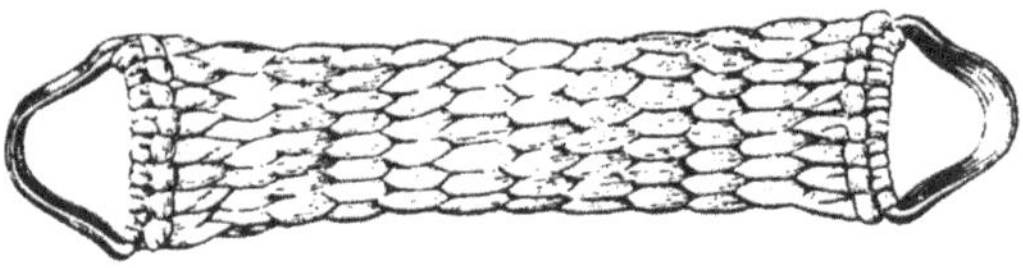

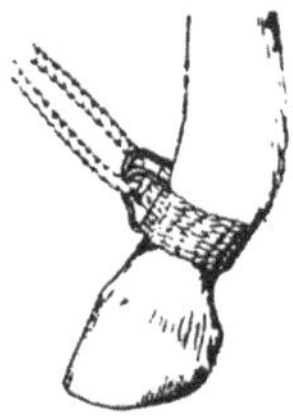

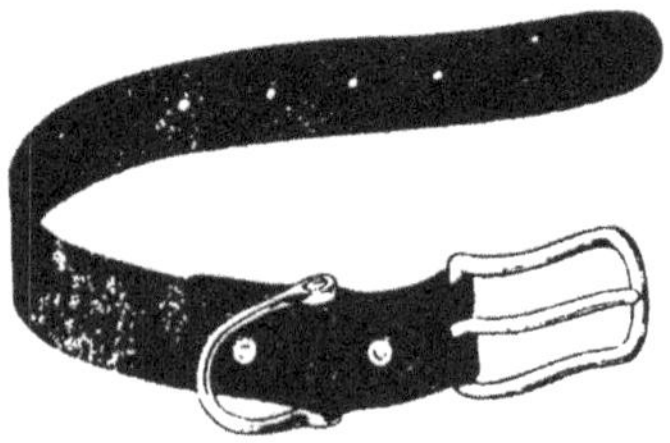

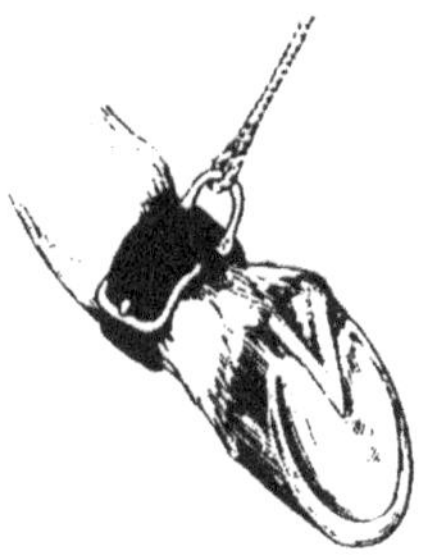

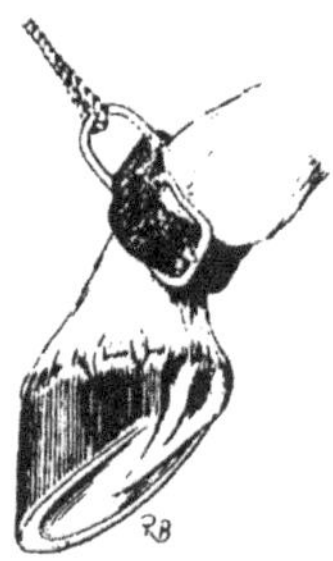

Temporary Rope Halter

The temporary halter may be used when a permanent halter is not available. If the lead rope is knotted securely at the throat so that the nose piece will not "draw down", it may, however, be used permanently.

- Loop the rope around the horse's neck and secure the loop with a bowline knot. (fig. 2.17)

- Make a bight in the standing part. (fig. 2.18)

- Pass the bight through the loop and over the horse's nose. (fig. 2.19)

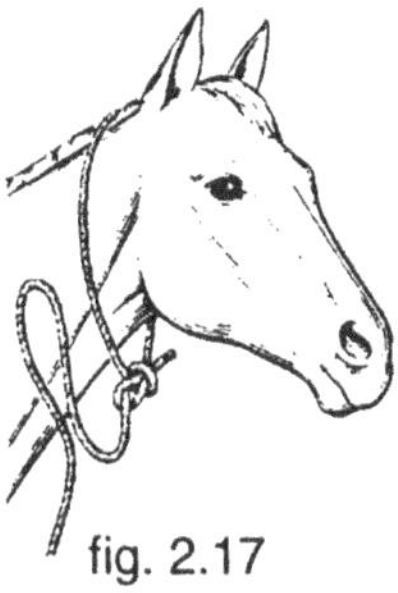

fig. 2.17

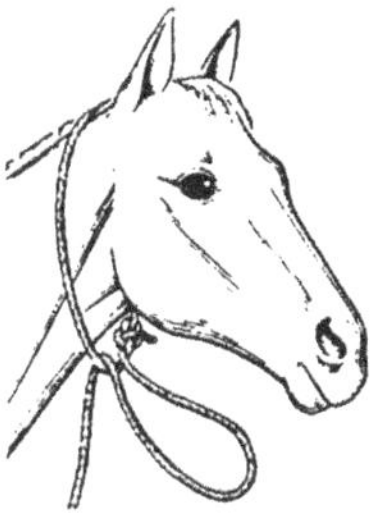

fig. 2.18

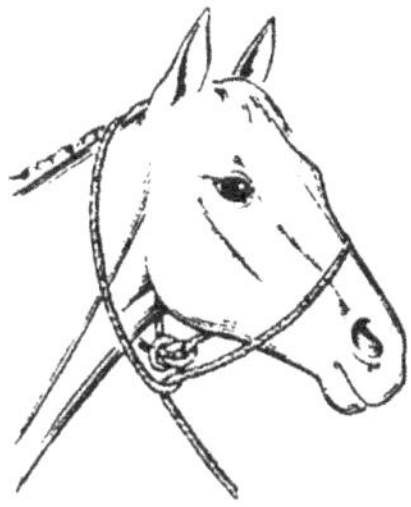

fig. 2.19

Yankee War Bridle

The war bridle is a simple type of restraint and when applied with judgment, is neither cruel nor harmful. The principle which makes it effective is, as with the twitch, that pain in one area diverts the horse's attention from another.

Ten feet of 5/6 or 3/8 inch rope are needed. An eye is formed in one end and the other passed through it to make a loop about three feet in diameter. The loop is placed so that it passes over the poll, down on both sides of the face and across the gum of the upper incisor teeth. It is convenient to have the eye with the end through it located as it is in the illustration. When the end is pulled, pressure is put on the poll and the gums causing pain to the horse.

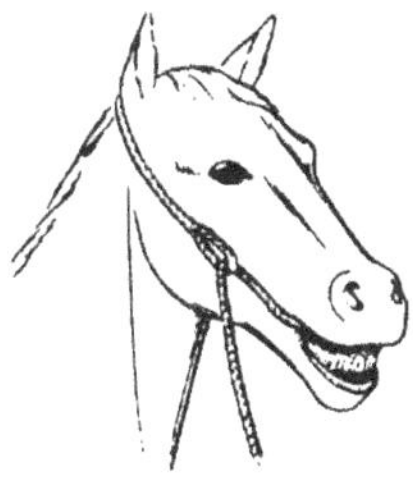

Hippo-harness

The hippo-harness is a good restraint for an animal that is obstreperous and likely to rear. The harness ropes cross over the withers and rump and by keeping the ropes taut one can apply enough pressure at these two points to keep the animal down. The harness permits some freedom of movement to the legs and for this reason is not a good one to prevent kicking. But many animals, for some reason, have their minds more on rearing than on kicking, and it is for a creature of this sort that a hippo-harness is intended.

A rope is thrown across the animal's back with its center at the withers. The ends are passed around the front legs, from the inside out to make a half hitch, and then carried back to the rear legs where the same process is repeated. Finally, they are crossed over the rump and held by assistants. The handlers should not stand directly behind the animal, but should stand at his flanks.

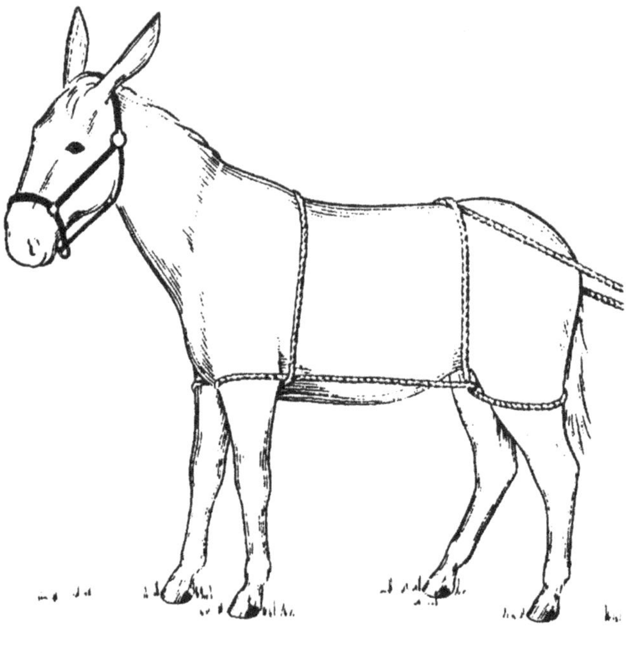

Double Side-line Casting Harness

The double side-line casting harness is the most practical method of casting a horse and restraining him in the recumbent position. It gives a maximum of restraint without special equipment, only two pieces of thirty foot rope or one sixty foot piece being required. If web hobbles are used, as illustrated, they will lessen the chance of rope burns on the animal's pasterns.

Double a sixty foot rope or tie together two thirty foot pieces. Form a rope collar that fits around the horse's chest, shoulders and withers. A bowline on the a bight is a convenient knot to use in forming a single strand rope collar which can be passed over the horse's head and fitted in position. A square or bowline knot can be used to form a double strand collar in position around the horse's shoulders. The ends of the rope should leave the collar at the withers, pass down, one on each side of the body, and go through both rings of a web hobble that has been placed on the pastern of the rear leg of that side. Take the end of the rope on each side forward again to the shoulder and pass it, from back to front, beneath the collar.

The end of the rope on the side on which the horse is to be cast is carried forward and held by one or two men. The end of the rope on the opposite side is carried backward, around the rump and away so that it forms a right angle with the long axis of the horse's body. One man holds this rope. The ropes must be held free of slack but without tension, or the horse will tread around in an effort to free his legs of the pastern hobbles. One man holds the halter rope, which may be passed over the horse's head, at the poll, for leverage when pulled toward the side on which the horse is to fall. (figs. 2.20 & 2.21)

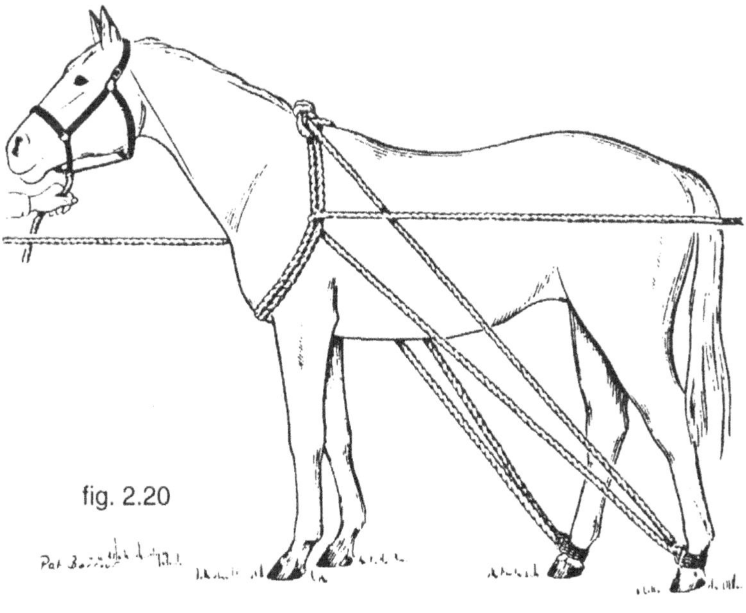

fig. 2.20

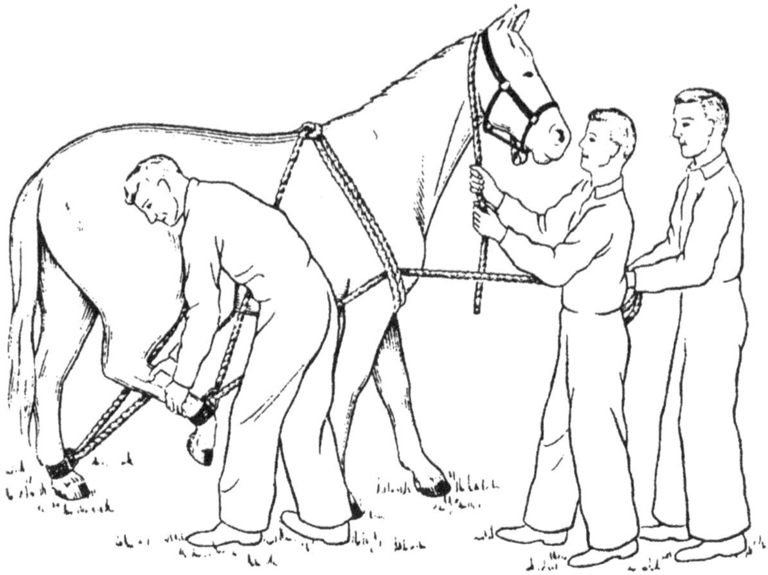

fig. 2.21

Casting: As one man raises the rear leg of the side on which the horse is to fall, the rope on that side is drawn tight to hold the leg in the raised position (fig. 2.21). The man who raises the leg moves clear of the horse, all the ropes are pulled simultaneously and the horse is thrown to the ground (fig. 2.22). The man holding the halter rope prevents the horse from raising his head and arranges the bedding beneath it. Both the casting ropes are held tight, and the man holding the upper one moves up to the horse's croup in readiness to tie the rear leg.

Alternate Method: The halter rope is not passed over the poll as illustrated. Instead, the man holding it grasps it close to its attachment and with it forces the horse backward into the harness. As the horse lifts his legs in moving back, tension is maintained on the casting ropes. The horse automatically falls in the direction of the stress on the rope around his rump. In this method of casting the position of the men is as illustrated (fig. 2.20).

With the upper casting ropes, the upper rear leg is flexed against the abdomen and a loop is thrown around the pastern from front to back. (fig. 2.23)

Tying is continued by passing the rope backward diagonally across the cannon bone, then across the medial side of the hock and around the hock to the lateral side. (fig. 2.24)

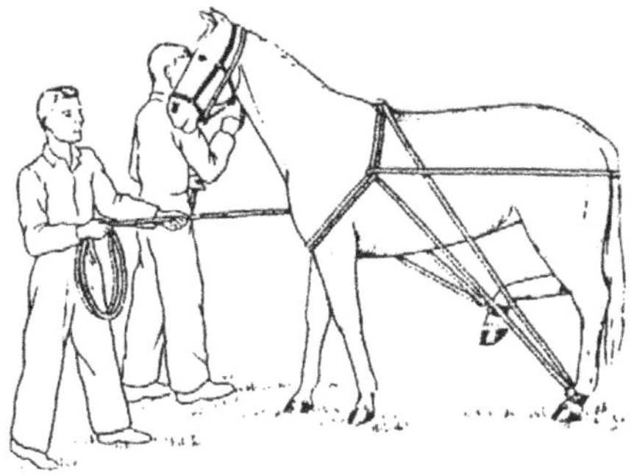

fig. 2. 22

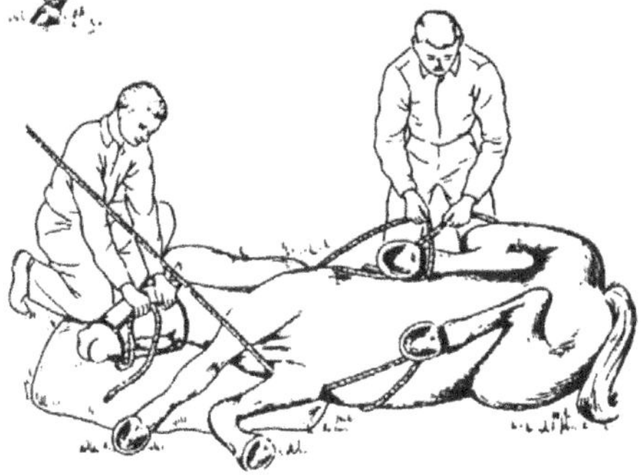

fig. 2.23

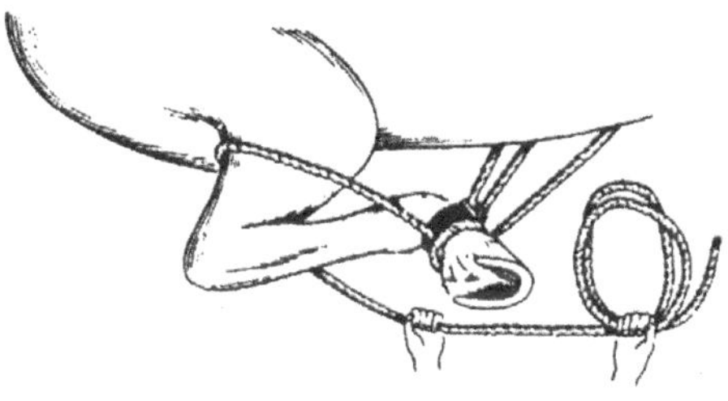

fig. 2.24

Pass the rope forward from the hock across the back of the cannon bone to the medial side of the pastern; then around the front of the pastern to the lateral side. Continue with the tying of the leg until two "figure 8's" have been completed and the rope is at the lateral side of the pastern. Form a bight in the rope. (fig. 2.25)

Pass the bight down between the ropes around the hock and the hock joint. Draw all the free end of the rope through the eye of the bight. Pull tight. (fig. 2.26)

Still pulling tightly on the end of the rope, straddle the neck of the horse and face his body. With the left hand flex the front leg and with the right hand throw a half hitch around the pastern. Pull the rope so that it draws the hoof of the front leg against the body and close to the hoof of the rear leg. (fig. 2.27)

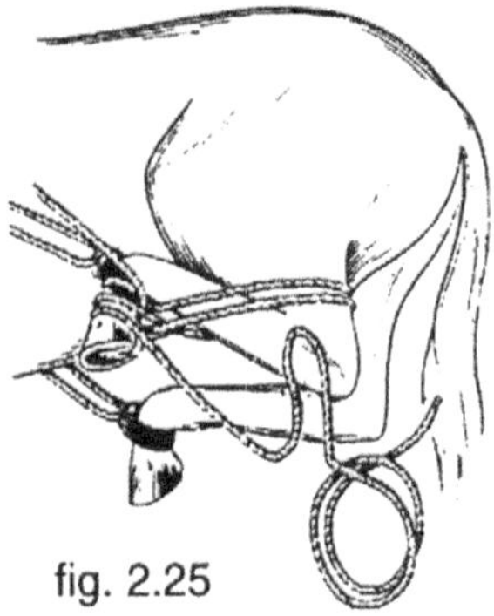

fig. 2.25

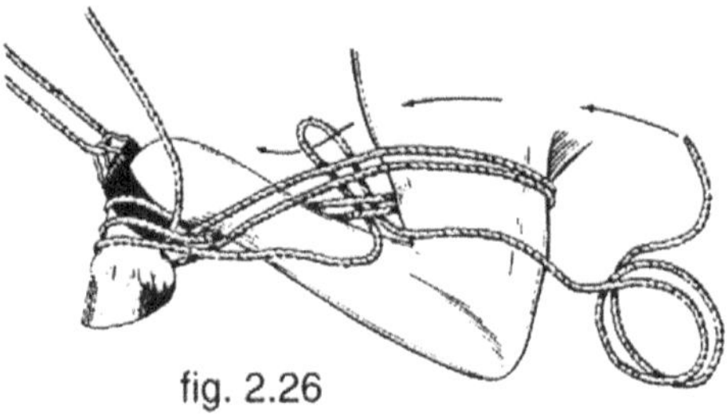

fig. 2.26

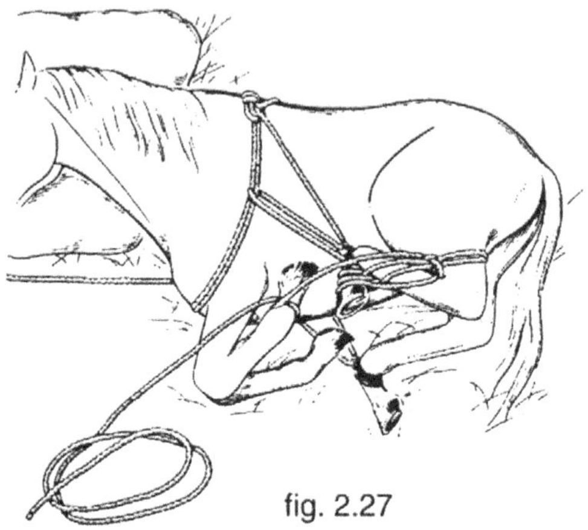

fig. 2.27

Form a half hitch in the rope and throw it over the flexed front leg. (figs. 2.28 & 2.29)

Throw another half hitch around the flexed front leg and draw the rope tight. (fig. 2.30)

These illustrations, for the sake of clarity, do not show the leg in complete flexion as it should be when tied.

Carry the end of the rope over to the ropes that pass from the collar to the rear leg and tie it securely. (fig. 2.31)

Continue to hold tight the rope which is beneath the horse. The man holding the head should shift his position, but continue to hold the head while the horse is rolled over and tied on the opposite side in a similar manner. (fig. 2.32)

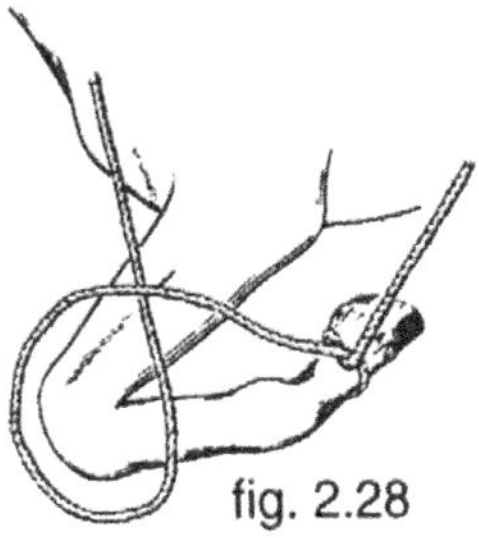
fig. 2.28

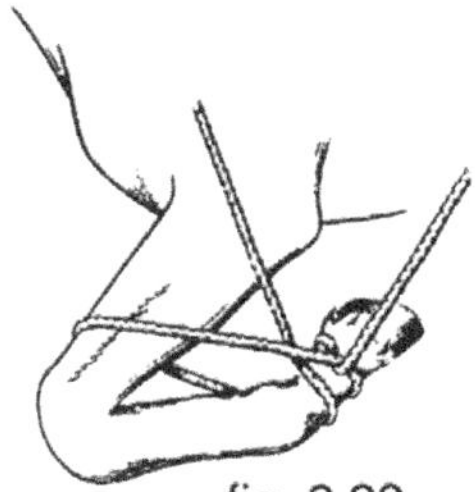
fig. 2.29

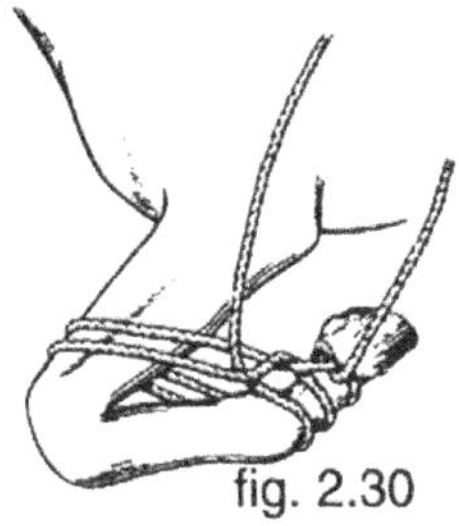
fig. 2.30

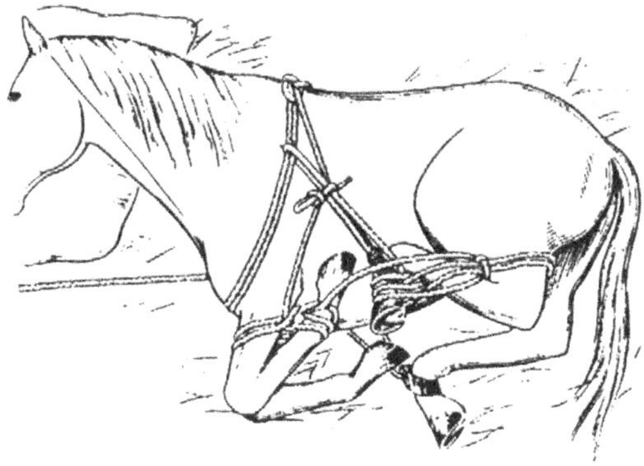
fig. 2.31

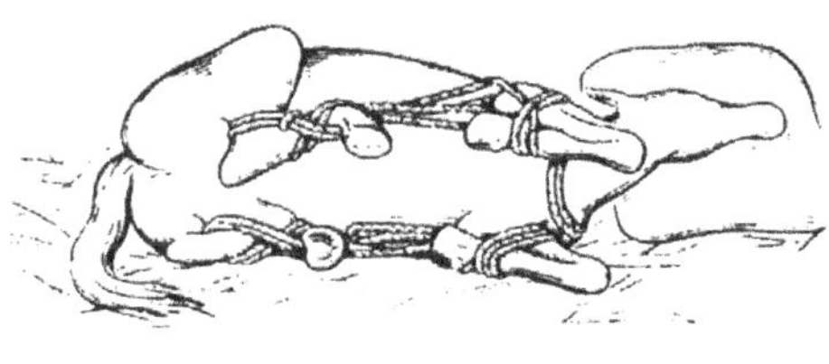
fig. 2.32

COW RESTRAINT

Although cattle do not show the individual differences that horses or pigs do, it is still quite an art to handle these animals. One has ample opportunity to exercise his knowledge of animal psychology by differentiating between the nervous cow, the docile cow, the balker and the chronic kicker. It is true, however, that cows do not respond to argument or reasoning as much as horses and pigs do. Usually they must be urged to do ones bidding.

There are some things which must be kept in mind in dealing with cattle. In the first place, dairy bulls should never be trusted. They often appear to be gentle and calm, particularly when they have been receiving regular attention from handlers. They are unpredictable, however, and it is a mistake to rely on what may appear to be their good nature. Whenever one is working with them, one should be sure to have them completely restrained. Beef bulls are not apt to be as mean and angry as dairy bulls, but they are far from gentle and should be handled carefully.

Whenever beef cattle are to be restrained standing they should be placed in a press or stocks. These animals are too large and strong to be easily restrained with ropes alone.

Dairy cows should be restrained as little as possible. They are used to being handled but they are excitable animals and fear the unusual. Hence they will often be upset by complicated restraints and resist them, but will submit rather calmly to simple things. Also, a cow's tail is not nearly as strong as a horse's, and these animals should never be pulled or dragged by their tails. Their caudal vertebrae could very easily be dislocated by this.

Cows who are kept in dark barns are apt to be nervous. The veterinarian who steps into such a barn, therefore, should be more on his guard than he would be if he were in a well lighted, well ventilated one.

Finally, anesthesia should accompany restraint in the more painful operations. The older custom was to rely solely on ropes and other restraints to hold an animal still while an operation was being done. As cows are particularly susceptible to pain, it is only humane, as well as practical, to use some sedative or anesthetic to keep a cow from struggling unnecessarily.

Restraints That Divert the Attention

These restraints, like the twitches, cause temporary pain in one place and thus take the animal's attention from other areas.

Tail Restraint

The tail restraint may be applied by an assistant whenever it is necessary to distract a cow's attention from another part of her body on which work is being done. It may be used when giving udder injections to a nervous cow. The assistant should keep both hands close to the base of the tail or he may break it. He should stand to one side of the cow to avoid being kicked. (fig. 2.33)

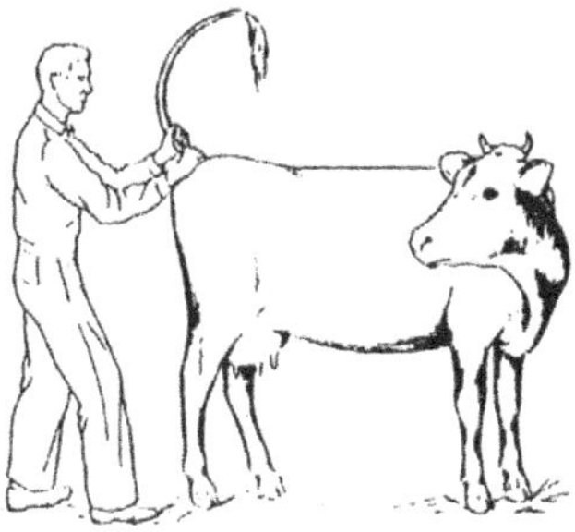

fig. 2.33

Hock Twitch

This twitch will prevent a cow from raising the rear leg and thus prevents kicking. It is a simple and effective restraint. It is made from a piece of heavy cotton rope between 18 and 22 inches long with an eye in both ends. The rope is placed around the animal's leg just above the hock joint and a strong stick or a piece of pipe about a foot long is put through each eye. By turning the stick one may twist the rope until it binds the leg tightly and presses the Achilles tendon down. Thus it prevents the animal's raising its leg and makes kicking impossible.(fig. 2.34)

Squeeze Restraint for Kicking

Another restraint that will keep a cow from kicking is that drawn below.

With a rope which has an eye in one end, a loop is formed around the cow's body in front of the udder. When the end is pulled tight so that the rope squeezes the cow, she will stand still. (fig. 2.35)

Dehorning Restraint

This restraint is a simple one but it will hold a cow's neck firmly. It may be used in a pasture for dehorning or in a corral or sales stable for making a quick examination for soundness. (figs. 2.36, 2.37 & 2.38)

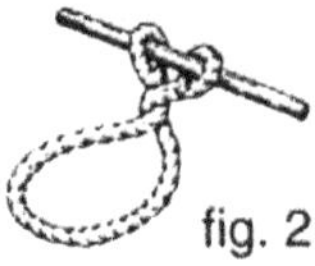

fig. 2.34

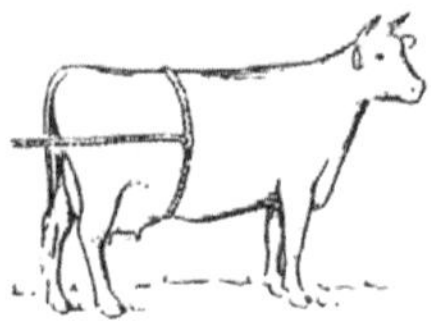

fig. 2.35

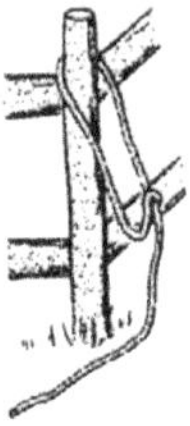

fig. 2.36

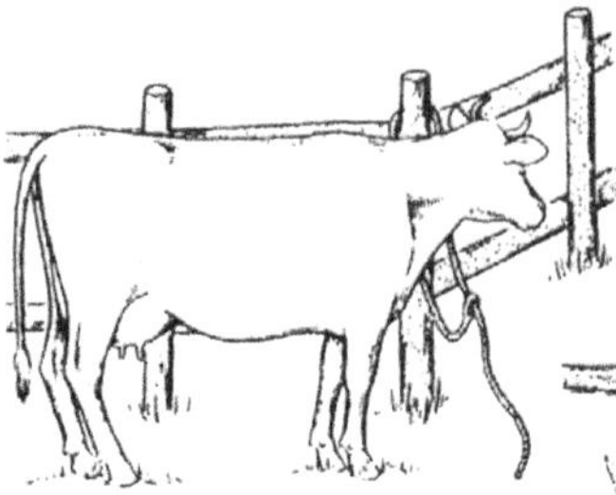

fig. 2.37

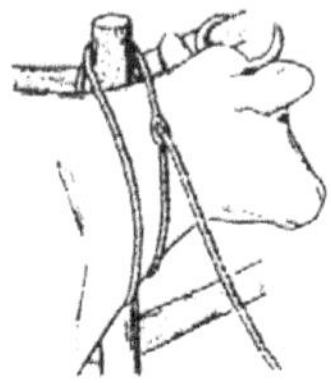

fig. 2.38

Casting Restraints

Cows are more easily and safely cast than horses since they struggle less and are more willing to lie down. Bedding should be arranged for them none the less, as it may save them from bruises.

Bulls are more vigorous and are harder to cast and control. It may be safer to cast them with a double side-line harness than with one of the squeezes.

Burley Method of Casting*

This method of casting cattle, devised by Dr. D. R. Burley of Georgia, has many advantages over the other casting methods. First, it is not necessary in this method to tie the rope around the horns or the neck. It is simply passed around the animal's body which takes less time. Second, this restraint does not put pressure over the thorax and thus does not interfere with the action of the heart and lungs. Third, it does not endanger the genital organs of the bull or the mammary vessels of the cow. Finally, with this restraint both rear legs may be tied with the ends of the casting rope.

While the cow is being held by a strong halter or by a nose lead a forty foot piece of rope is placed over her back with its center at the withers. The ends are carried between the forelegs and crossed at the sternum. One end is carried up each side of the animal's body and the two are crossed again over the back. Each end passes downward between the rear legs going between the inner surface of the legs and the udder or scrotum, as the case may be. (figs. 2.39 & 2.40)

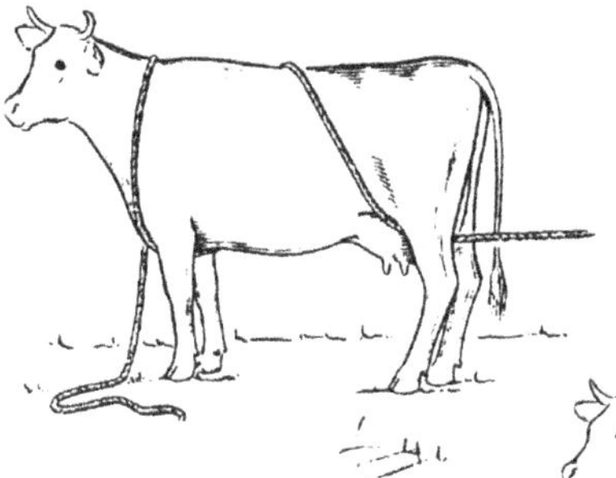

fig. 2.39

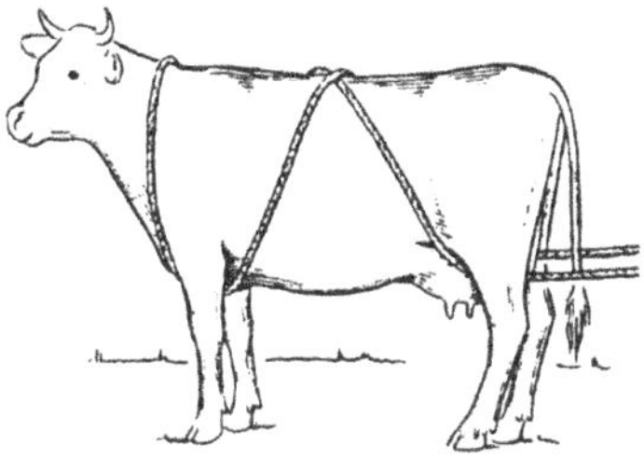

fig. 2.40

***Leard, T., and Leonard, C., "The Georgia Vet.", Univ. of Ga.**

When the ends of the rope are pulled, the cow will fall. The operator may control the direction of the fall by pulling the casting ropes so that the animal is forced to one side or the other.

To tie the rear leg, the operator keeps both ropes taut and slides the uppermost one along the under surface of the rear leg to the fetlock. He flexes the leg and makes a half hitch around the fetlock. (fig. 2.41)

The end is then carried around the leg above the hock, across the cannon bone, and back around the fetlock. The leg is secured by several such "figure 8's". (figs. 2.42 & 2.43)

To tie the front leg a short heavy cord or rope about six feet long is needed. One end of it is fastened around the pastern with a clove hitch leaving a free end about eight inches long. The front leg is flexed and the long end of the cord carried forward and passed under the main casting rope descending from the withers. (fig. 2.44)

The cord is passed around the flexed front leg several times and tied in a reefer's knot to the short free end at the pastern. (fig. 2.45)

The animal is rolled over and the rear leg of the other side tied with the other end of the casting rope. With another six foot cord, the other front leg is tied, and the animal is then completely restrained.

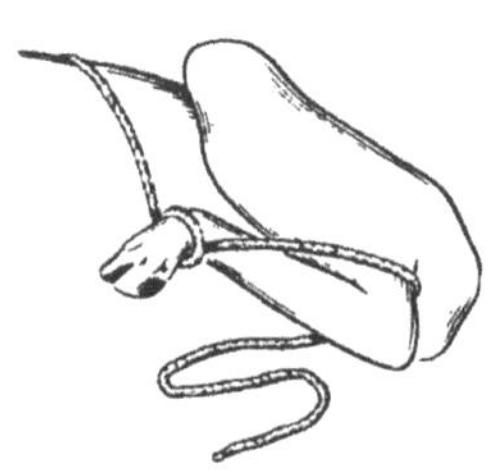

fig. 2.41

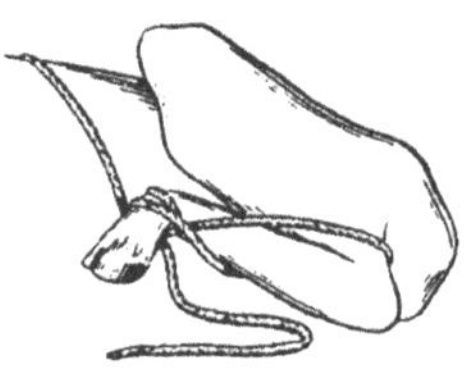

fig. 2.42

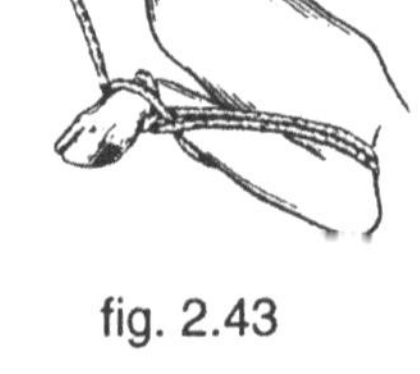

fig. 2.43

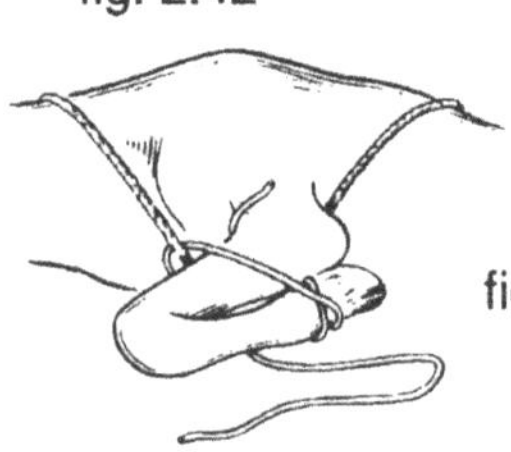

fig. 2.44

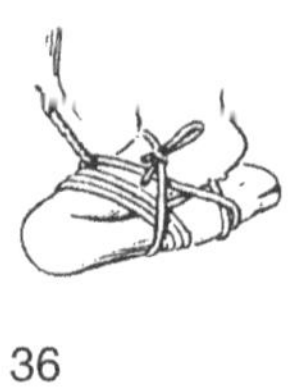

fig. 2.45

PIG RESTRAINT

There are some peculiarities about the build and temperament of pigs which those dealing with them should always keep in mind. They are stubborn and have definite ideas of their own and they are extreme individualists. "Pigs should be dealt with kindly. Few animals are more amenable to training"*

In spite of the pig's hardy appearance he is not athletic and cannot stand very rough handling, especially in hot weather. Also, his legs are thin and rather easily fractured. On the other hand, pigs are not gentle animals and many of them do not handle their attendants with too much kindness. Even a baby pig is capable of biting and the brute strength and tusks of a boar make him a menacing animal. A sow with piglings may be particularly cross and ill-natured.

A pig's eyes are deeply set and his body smooth, streamlined and tough, to enable him to work his way through dense thickets. His eyesight is not too keen, and for this reason he is easily frightened if not carefully maneuvered. It is instinctive for him to spot a small opening and head for it even though it is no larger than the space between the legs of a man who is trying to catch him. Because his body is so smooth, he is able to slip through one's hands and to elude catching.

It is very difficult to drive or pull pigs, as they usually want to go in the other direction. If they are roaming loose, they may be coaxed into a sty by the attendant who usually feeds them, or they may be made to enter by surrounding them with barriers which prevent their going anywhere else. One should never get into an enclosure or pen with a pig that may be vicious without first making sure that there is some way of escaping quickly.

Much may be done with some pigs by talking to them in a calm and soothing way or by scratching their backs or heads. With some pigs more can be accomplished by conversation or scratching than by ropes. If the animal is lying down, the veterinarian should approach it quietly, talk to it, and scratch it. Thus, he may be able to examine it thoroughly with no restraint whatever. In some cases he may rely on the owner who may have developed special ways of handling his animals.

When fairly painful or prolonged work is to be done and restraint is necessary, the veterinarian should attempt to make the animal as comfortable as possible and yet make quite sure that he remains in the original position and under control until released. Because of a pig's strength complete restraint is difficult, but it is necessary.

When a large number of pigs are to be dealt with, it is advisable to have them as clean and dry as possible. Several days before they are to be handled, if there pen is cleaned and fresh bedding supplied, they will have a chance to dry off and will be easier to cope with.

Catching a Small Pig

When a little pig is to be caught he should be captured immediately and held firmly but comfortably. He should never be hunted or chased as this will frighten him unnecessarily and if repeated may lead to his developing a bad temper or nervous disposition.

To lift a pigling only a few days old, one should grab him quickly from behind, seizing one or both hind legs or gripping his body just behind the shoulders. He should then be held with one hand under his body and the other over his shoulders. (fig. 2.46) If he squeals, he should be taken where the sow and other pigs cannot hear him as his cries will upset them.

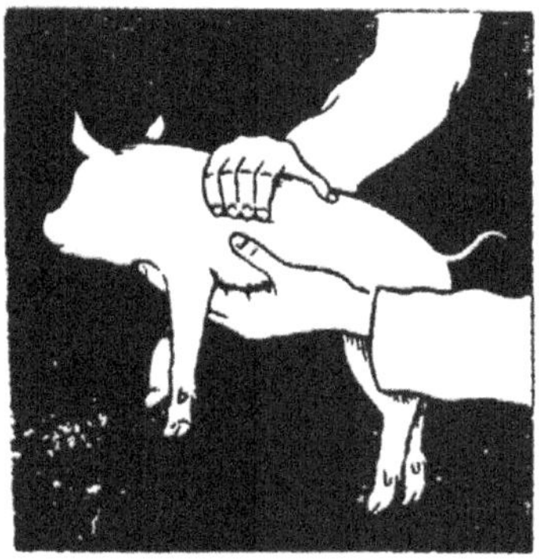

fig. 2.46

***Davidson, H. R., "The Production and Marketing of Pigs", London, 1948, p. 388.**

One ought never to lift or to hold a pigling by his ears or tail. Many stockmen do this, but it is a bad practice. A pig's ears and tail are sensitive and pulling on them is painful to him. He will squirm to get out of his handler's grasp, if he is held in this manner and if he is wet and slippery he may succeed.

On the other hand, if he is lifted quickly by the hind legs and held firmly around the body, he will be much easier to hold. He will be frightened at first, but as he is being held comfortably, he will calm down quickly.

Catching a Large Pig

A large pig who has been maneuvered into a pen or some such limited space can be caught with a snare or with a rope. It is futile to try to catch big pigs with the bare hands as their bodies are naturally so smooth and usually so slippery that they can easily slip out of one's grasp. With the following method they can be quite simply caught and held.

A large loop formed from a rope with an eye in one end is flung around the pig's neck. (fig. 2.47) As soon as his neck is caught in the noose, the pig's movements will become unpredictable. He may move in any direction and the handler must be alert and ready for the time when he is about to go forward.

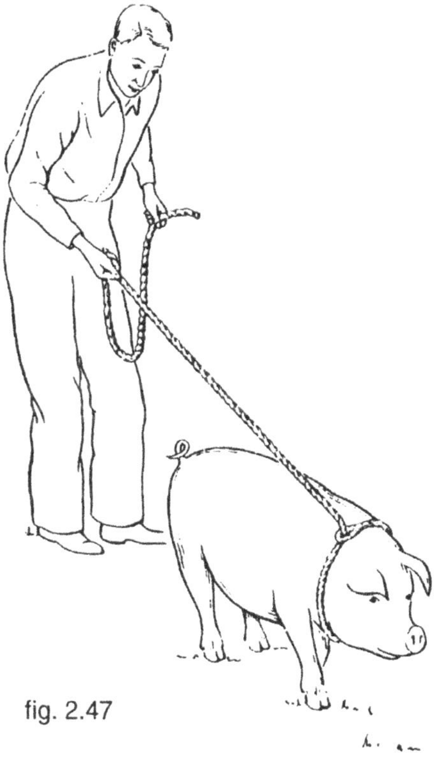

fig. 2.47

Holding firmly to the end of the rope he quickly throws the standing part on the ground in front of the pig so that he will step over it as he tries to run away. As he does this, he should stand behind the animal for the psychology of the pig is such that he will go forward to escape a man behind him. (fig. 2.48)

The end is passed under the standing part to form a half hitch around the pig's body. (fig. 2.49)

Some may prefer to form the half hitch in the rope first and hold the loop in front of the pig so that he runs through it. (fig. 2.50)

As the pig tries to escape, pull tight. (fig. 2.51)

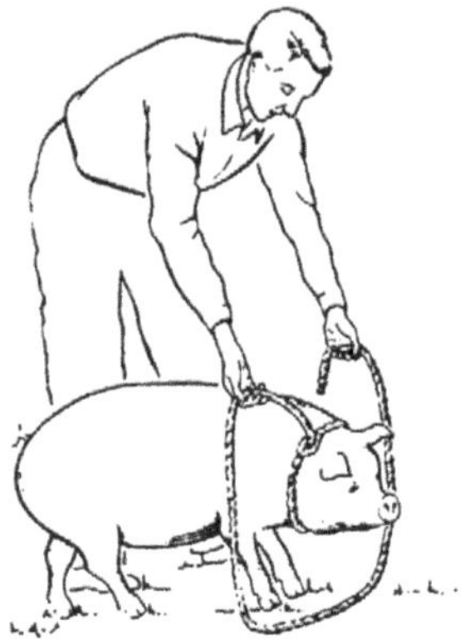

fig. 2.48

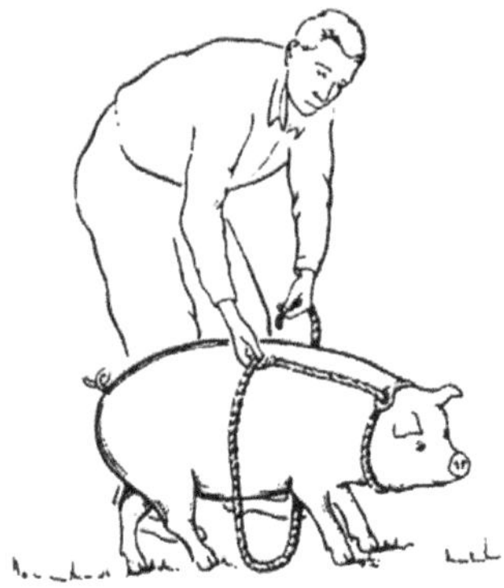

fig. 2.49

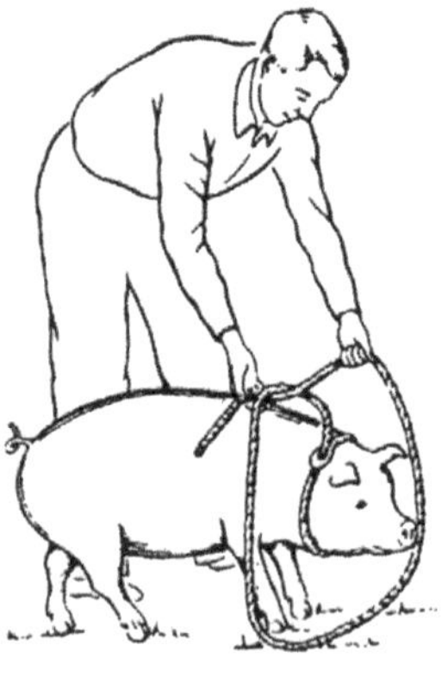

fig. 2.50

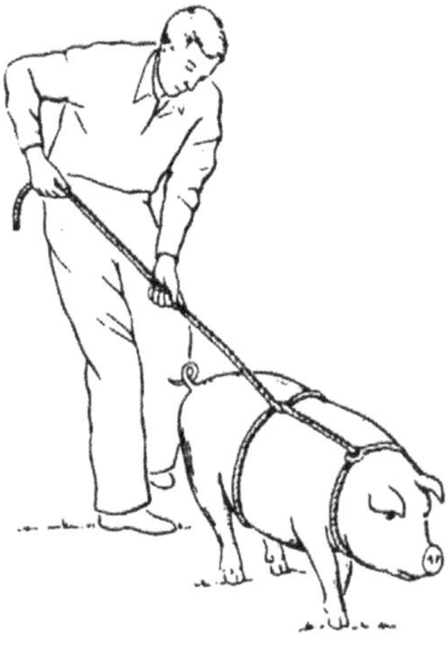

fig. 2.51

Snubbing Rope

After the pig is caught or confined in close quarters, this head tie may be used to make him easier to handle or to tie him to a fixed object.

With a 10 foot piece of rope which has an eye in one end a loop is made. If the pig is "ringed" he may fear anything near his snout and in this case a large loop will be needed. Standing behind the pig, the handler places the loop over his nose. If, within a few moments the pig does not become curious and open his mouth, the handler can pull the rope with a sawing motion from side to side against the upper jaw and force the pig's mouth open. The loop should then be pushed quickly into the mouth behind the tusks and tightened. (fig. 2.52)

An assistant may hold the rope and stand directly in front of the pig. (fig. 2.53) His presence will cause the animal to pull back and this is quite often sufficient restraint for vaccination, clipping tusks, oral dosing or treating body wounds. If the nose is snubbed to something close to the ground so that he is unable to crouch down, a mature boar may even be castrated with only this restraint.

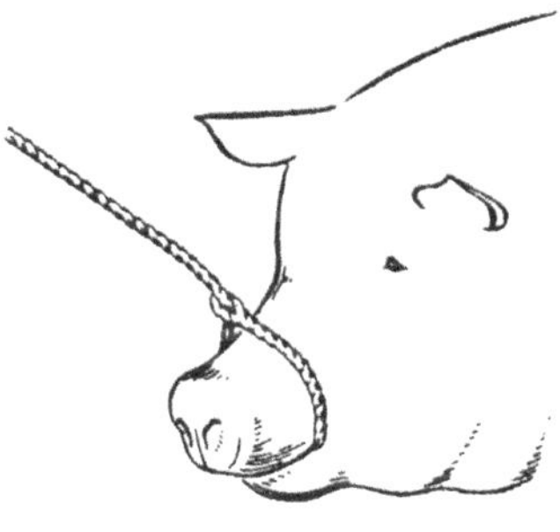

fig. 2.52

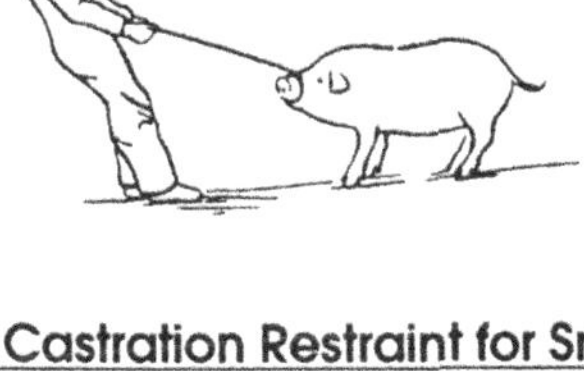

fig. 2.53

Vaccination or Castration Restraint for Small Pigs

A pig under a hundred pounds in weight may be held by the hind legs with his body, ventral surface forward, gripped between the assistant's knees and his head downward. This is a simple way to restrain a pig for vaccination. (fig. 2.54) For castration, the pig may be turned so that his back is forward and his head passes between the assistant's legs. (fig. 2.55) These restraints require a strong and untiring handler. When a drove of pigs is to be treated, he should stand near a gate or door that can be opened to allow each pig to pass through as he is released. If the pig is held so that his front feet rest on the ground, he will struggle less and some of his weight will be supported.

Vaccination or Worming Restraint for Large Pigs

Usually a pig holder, obstetrical snare or a snubbing-rope will restrain a big pig sufficiently so that he may be injected in back of the ears or in one of the forelegs. If, for some reason, it is preferred to vaccinate him in the axillary or inguinal spaces, a large pig may be set back on his haunches and held by the forelegs with his body wedged between the knees of the assistant. (fig. 2.56) Being held in this peculiar position usually unnerves a pig so much that he will become more tractable than he ordinarily might be. For giving capsules one might hold a pig in this way and use a balling-gun, or for giving liquids a speculum and stomach tube could be used.

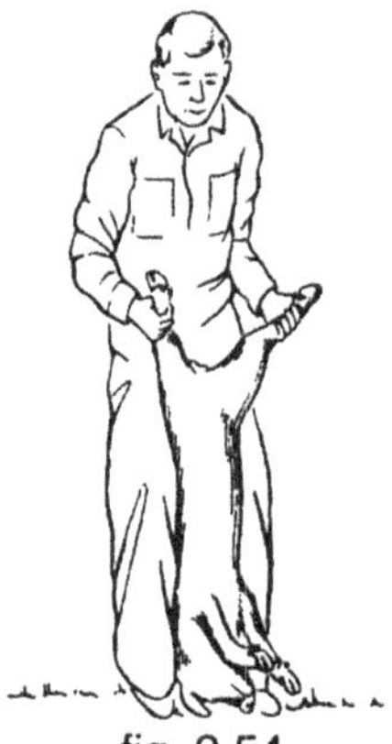

fig. 2.54

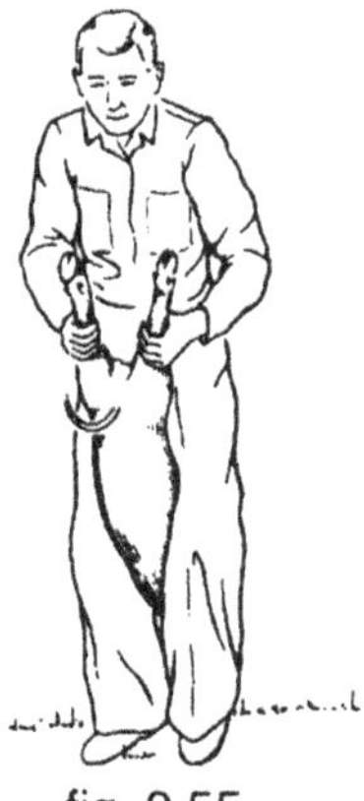

fig. 2.55

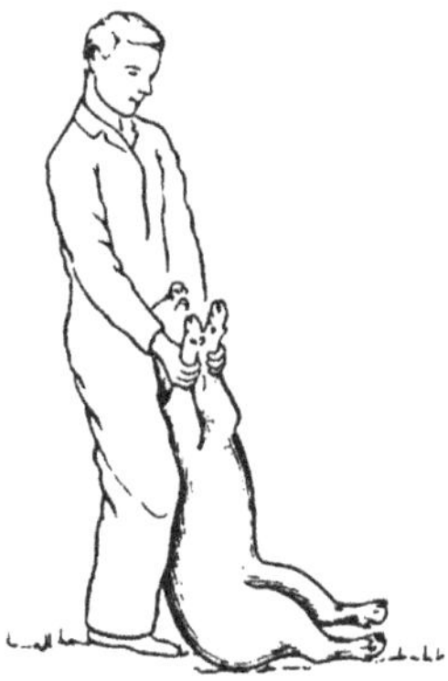

fig. 2.56

Restraint of a Pig in a Trough

On most farms where there are pigs there is usually to be found a trough of some kind. Such a trough may be useful for holding a pig in almost any position. If assistants are available they may hold the pig in the trough or he may be fastened by a rope which passes from one leg around the outside of the trough to a leg of the opposite side. The trough may then be tilted against a fence or some other stationary object so that the pig is held with either head or hind end up, as is preferred. (fig, 2.57)

Casting Restraint

For this restraint the pig should be tied with a snubbing rope. To cast him on his right side, the end of the snubbing rope is carried back to the left hind leg and passed around it, above the hock, from the inside out. (fig. 2.58)

When all is in readiness for the pig to fall, the end of the rope is pulled, thus drawing the hock close to the head and throwing the pig off balance. The rope should be pulled tight when the pig is down, and the end passed under the standing part to be secured by a half hitch. (fig. 2.59)

Instead of passing the rope around the leg, one may place a hobble around it and let the rope go through its ring. As the legs have much freedom of movement in this restraint, it is suitable only for work of short duration, unless the pig is also given some anesthesia. Also, an assistant could hold the bottom leg firmly by standing with his foot over it.

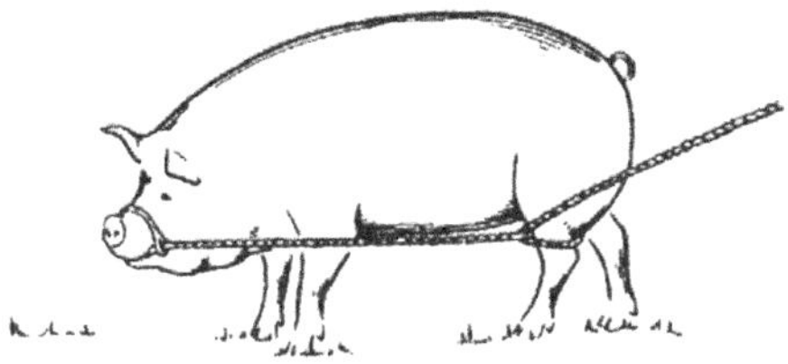

fig. 2.58

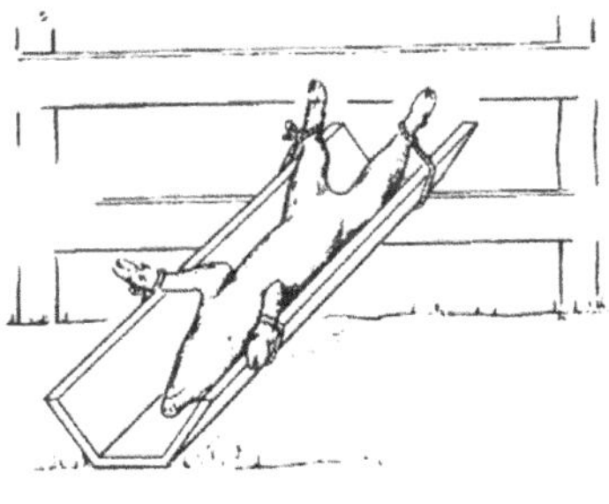

fig. 2.57

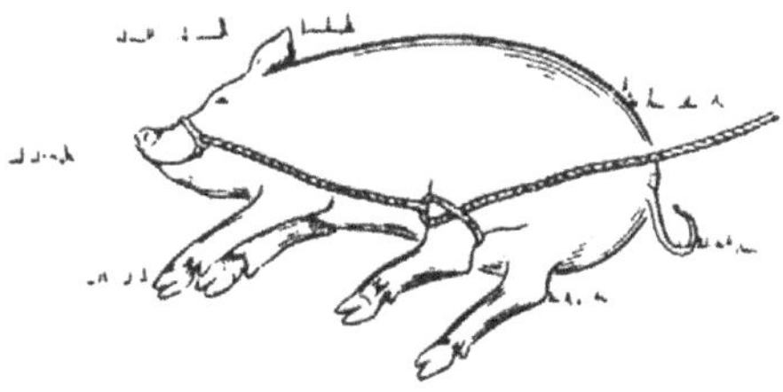

fig. 2.59

For doing prolonged work or work which requires cleaner conditions, the pig's legs should be bound together so that they will not stir up dirt. A rope may be passed in a "figure 8" around the pastern of a hind leg and the front leg of the same side. Two, three or all four of the pig's legs may be bound together in this way and an anesthetic given for complete restraint. (fig. 2.60)

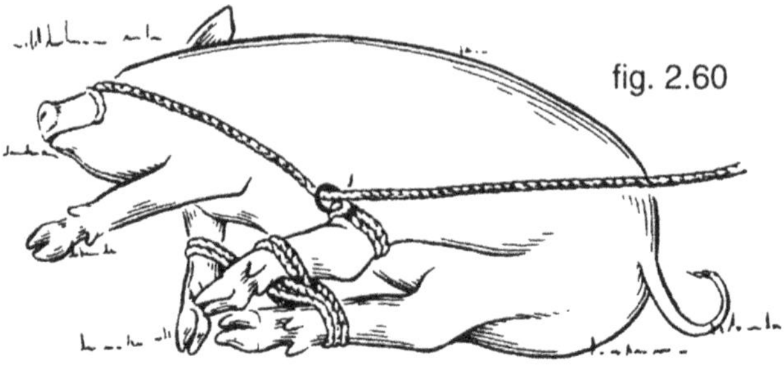

fig. 2.60

Casting Restraint, Second Method

When the pig is secured with a holder or snubbing rope, he is led up to a fence or other barrier to which he can be fastened. Short ropes are looped around the front and rear legs of the side next to the fence. The end of the rope from the rear foot is carried forward under his body over his shoulder and around a post at his head. The rope from the front foot is passed under the body across the ham and then around a post at the tail.

When the two ropes are pulled tight, the pig will fall. If they are tied to the posts down close to the pig's body, they will hold him down quite effectively. (fig. 2.61)

If complete restraint is necessary for the particular work to be done, the pig's legs should be tied together.

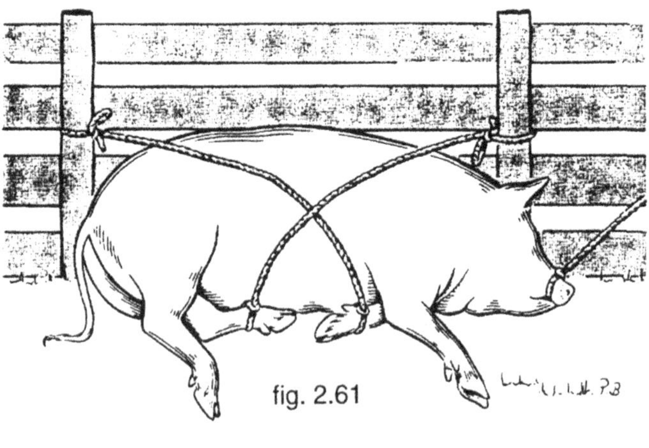

fig. 2.61

SHEEP RESTRAINT

Anyone can learn to handle sheep, but some people seem to have a "knack" with the animals. In England there is a common saying that lame men are the best shepherds. This is probably because they are more likely to possess the steady, calm, patient type of personality that is needed for getting along well with sheep.

Sheep are spoken of as timid, nervous animals that are easily frightened. This is true of the sheep that are generally known and is largely due to the way they are kept. They are kept in large bands away from people and other animals as beef cattle are and for this reason develop a similar wild, nervous temperament. When one compares the temperament of a beef breed cow with that of a cow of the same breed kept in a dairy herd, he finds a difference comparable to that between a sheep raised in a flock and one raised as a cosset. Handling can do much to tame sheep as is evidenced by those in France and the Balkan countries that are raised for milking and cheese making. These sheep are as quiet and steady as the average dairy cow.

Sheep differ from most other domesticated animals in that they have little means of defense other than butting, stamping their forefeet or running away from their adversary. Their usual defense is to run, and in so doing they may totally exhaust themselves as very often happens when strange dogs approach. Dogs do more harm in entertaining themselves by chasing a flock of sheep than they do by the actual killing of a few. In order to give their sheep a feeling of security and to provide an example of courage, some owners keep a goat or two with their flocks. The sheep will be less likely to flee if they see a goat stand his ground. This arrangement works very well if the goats are brought up with the flock from the time they are kids. Fully grown goats placed suddenly in a flock, however, quickly become bored and wander off from the sheep.

When working with sheep one must think not of possible danger to himself, as he would when working with a horse, bull or vicious dog, but one must consider the damage that may be done to the animal in the struggle to catch and hold him. Sheep have a frail skeletal system; their legs and backs can easily be broken. Patches of wool can be pulled out readily and little effort is required to tear their skin.

Excitement must always be avoided in any activities where sheep are involved. It is a good idea to talk to the creatures or to whistle when approaching them in order that they will not be startled. It does little good, however, to attempt to reason with a sheep as one would with a horse or a dog. Sheep, unlike pigs, do not appreciate having their backs scratched nor do they respond favorably to petting as a horse or a dog will. Horses and dogs are handled individually, and their different personalities must be taken into account. Sheep, on the contrary, are usually handled as members of a flock, and for this reason any mistake in handling them is greatly multiplied. One upset animal can cause terror to sweep rapidly through a whole flock, and the resulting confusion can be chaotic. For a handler to deal successfully with these animals, gentleness, calmness and assurance are absolutely necessary.

A shepherd's crook may be used to catch one or more sheep from a flock without the aid of an enclosure. When a crook is used it should be hooked around the sheep's hind leg just above the hock. If the leg is caught below the hock, it may be broken. A handler can also grasp a sheep's leg at this place with his hands. The preferred way to catch a sheep by hand, however, is to place an arm around his jaw and around his neck.

One ought never to catch a sheep by his wool. This pulls and blemishes the wool and always leaves a bruise or black mark on the body which will diminish the value of the carcass.

To hold a sheep stand on the animal's left side. Place the left hand under his jaw and the right arm around behind his thighs. The left arm will prevent his moving forward and the right arm around his back, will stop backward movement.

Do not attempt to keep a sheep from moving by pulling on his head, horns or wool. He will quickly become excited and resist this. Merely keep a gentle pressure with the hand under his jaw.

Shearing and Hoof-trimming Restraint

In order that the wool can be kept clean, the sheep to be clipped should be placed on a smooth board platform about ten feet square. Animals waiting their turn should be kept in a clean pen so that they will not drag manure or litter with them into the shearing place.

There are several unnecessarily brutal methods of restraining sheep for clipping. It is the custom in some regions to tie the animal's front and hind legs to a board so that he cannot kick. This method is time consuming for the operator and very hard on the sheep. All experienced sheep owners object to it. In their haste to clip as many animals as fast as possible, some shearers keep hold of the shearing shaft and throw each successive sheep by grasping his back leg and giving him a vicious swing. This type of handling should not be tolerated, particularly if there are pregnant ewes in the flock.

To restrain a sheep correctly, the shearer, if right handed, stands to the sheep's left, puts the left arm around his neck at the shoulder points and passes his right arm under the animal to grasp his right rear leg. He gently lifts him off his feet and sets him on his rump with his back toward him. The whole secret of successful restraint is in the adjustment of this position. The sheep's body should be tilted at an angle back toward the legs of the handler so that he is off balance and helpless. If his legs are unable to make sufficient contact with the floor, he will be unable to offer effective resistance and will not kick or struggle. With the animal in such a position the shearer can quite easily hold him securely with his left arm and have his right hand free for clipping.

Sheep should be held this same way for hoof-trimming or for vaccination in the groin where the wool-free skin is.

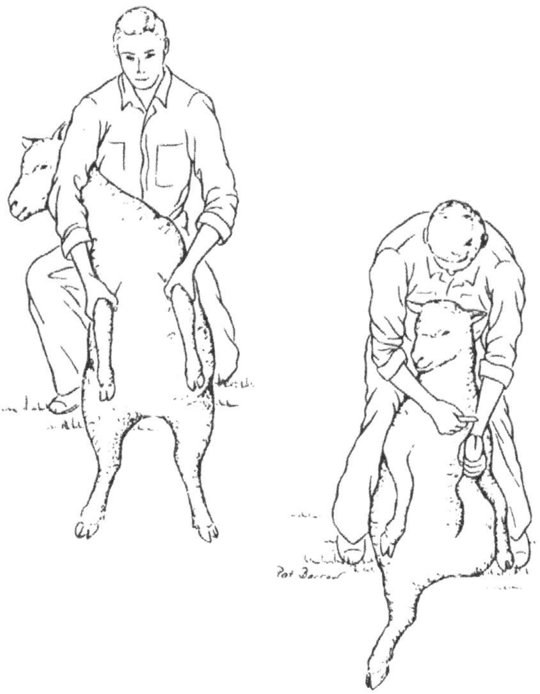

Castration Restraint

To avoid extra handling, lambs are usually castrated and docked at the same time. This should be done when they are between one and two weeks old. They should be put in a clean dry pen a day before in order that they can be caught easily, one at a time without being chased or excited before the operations. The castration should be done only on a bright clear day - never when it is damp or chilly.

To restrain a lamb for castration the assistant holds his two right legs in his right hand, his left ones in the left hand and supports his back between his legs. After the operation, the lambs should be returned to a clean, dry pen.

Sheep are quite susceptible to tetanus, and the veterinarian should take every precaution to protect himself and the animals at this time.

Tail Docking Restraint

Docking of sheep is most important as filth collects around the tail and in warm weather blow flies or screw worms may infest the area. Also, ewes with tails have trouble breeding.

Lambs between one and two weeks old are small enough for an assistant to hold comfortably. If the operator prefers to use a knife or an emasculator for docking, the assistant can stand holding the lamb's two right legs in his right hand, his two left legs in his left hand and the lamb's back against his body.

In using the Whitlock method, one should pen the sheep beforehand so that they are readily available. Several assistants are needed. One keeps the sheep moving along and does the marking. Another restrains the sheep so that the veterinarian is free to use both hands. This man straddles the animal and holds him firmly between his knees. He uses both hands to steady the sheep's head and to hold it so that the oral cavity is in line with the esophagus. The veterinarian faces the sheep and inserts the cannula of the syringe into the mouth and down the esophagus. It is almost impossible to insert the tube into the trachea. Thus, loss by inhalation of the drench into the lungs is negligible with this method of drenching. This is an excellent way to treat large flocks, for with good handing several hundred sheep can be drenched in an hour.

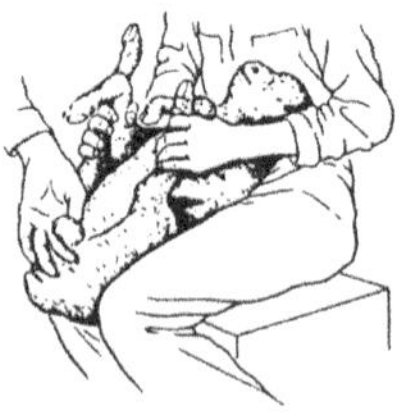

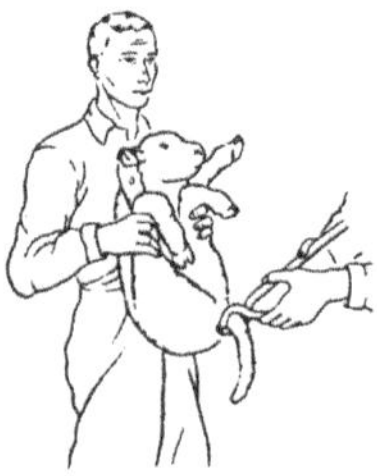

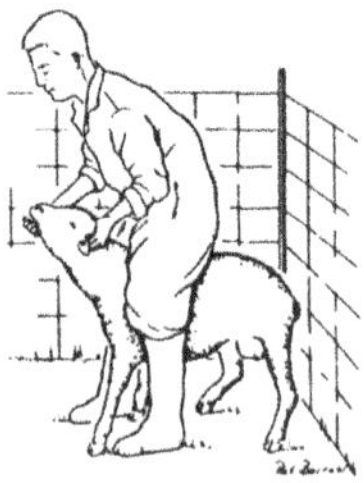

GOAT RESTRAINT

Unfortunately there is a widely prevailing belief that the goat is a robust, can-eating, elm-peeling scavenger that will thrive under the most adverse conditions with no care whatsoever. This notion is entirely erroneous. Goats are hardy creatures, but if they are to be raised profitably, they must be husbanded as carefully as any other domestic animal.

Goats suffer from many of the same ailments which plague sheep. They too must be dipped or sprayed, their hoofs must be trimmed and Angoras must be clipped. They are approximately the same size as sheep. For these reasons many of the restraint techniques used for sheep are also used for goats.

Any similarity between sheep and goats, however, applies only to some physical qualities and to size. In temperament and personality sheep and goats are as different as night and day.

Although many people keep a single doe for milk, this is not a good idea. Goats are not gregarious from fear or from a lack of personal resourcefulness as sheep are, but they truly suffer from loneliness. They like company for the pure pleasure of playing with other creatures. For this reason it is always better to have at least two goats. They are happier and easier to handle.

Of all creatures they are less easily subjugated to the human will, and they absolutely cannot be controlled by force alone. Fortunately, most goats are eager to establish loving relationships with their handlers, and this tendency should be encouraged. One who understands their varying moods can manage even the bucks quite easily through their quick and ardent affections. In fact, none of the herd are so affectionate by nature as the bucks. "Even a headstrong buck in a tremendous hurry to get to a waiting doe can be easily controlled by a firm grip on his beard and a tap on his nose with a small switch."* This, of course, is true only if the buck likes his handler.

Obviously, animals that are well bred and have been properly reared are easier to handle than those who have not. If a goat has been mistreated and improperly handled, his personality will reflect it. At any rate, whether an animal has been properly reared or not, a handler would be well advised not to insult a goat by turning his back on him. If he is not a close friend of the goat's, the temptation may be too great.

***Richards, I., Modern Milk Goats, Philad., J.B. Lippincott Co., 1921**

SECTION 3

DETERMINING DRUG DOSAGES

DETERMINING DOSAGES

ESTIMATING BODY WEIGHT

The first step in determining how much medicine an animal needs is to determine how much the animal weighs. Often a scale to weigh the larger animals is not available, but an accurate method of estimating weight uses a heart girth measurement. Heart girth is the distance around the animal's chest, measured just behind the front legs.

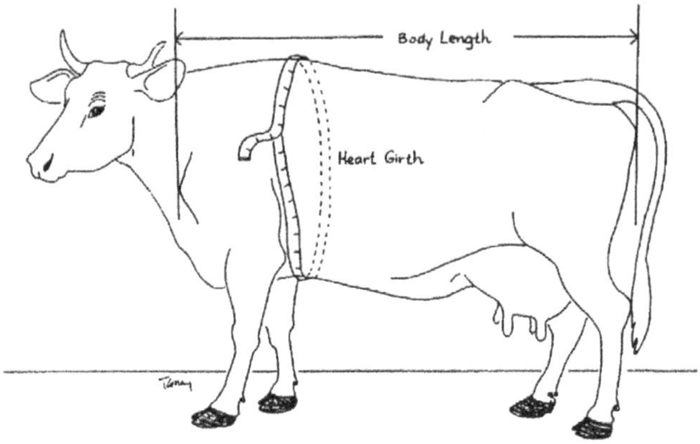

Cattle

To estimate weight on a cow, steer, or bull, measure the heart girth, then measure the body length. Body length is measured from the point of the shoulder (the most forward part of the shoulder) to the back of the pinbone (the bone to the side of the tail).

Use the numbers determined in the following formula:

$$\frac{\text{heart girth in cm} \times \text{heart girth in cm} \times \text{body length in cm}}{10{,}840} = \text{weight in kg}$$

Pigs

In pigs weight may be estimated using only the heart girth measurement, with the following formula:

$$\frac{\text{heart girth in cm} \times \text{heart girth in cm}}{120.6} = \text{weight in kg}$$

Goats

Use the following chart to determine weight after measuring the heart girth.

Heart Girth in Centimeters	Weight in Kilograms	Heart Girth in Centimeters	Weight in Kilograms
27.3	2.27	47.6	11.34
28.8	2.49	48.9	12.24
29.9	31.1	50.2	13.15
31.1	2.95	51.4	14.06
32.4	3.17	52.7	14.97
33.7	3.63	53.9	15.87
34.9	4.08	53.9	15.87
36.2	4.54	56.5	17.69
37.5	4.99	57.8	19.05
38.7	5.44	59.1	20.41
40.0	5.90	60.3	21.77
41.3	6.40	61.6	23.13
42.7	7.71	62.9	24.49
43.8	8.62	64.1	25.85
45.1	9.52	65.4	27.21
46.4	10.43	66.7	28.57
68.7	29.93	88.3	56.69
69.2	31.29	89.5	58.96
70.5	32.65	90.6	61.22
71.7	34.01	92.1	63.49
73.0	35.37	93.4	65.76
74.3	36.73	94.6	68.08
75.6	38.10	95.9	70.29
76.8	39.46	97.2	74.83
78.0	40.82	98.4	77.10
79.4	42.18	99.7	79.37
80.7	44.00	101.0	81.63
81.9	45.80	102.2	83.90
83.2	47.62	103.5	86.17
84.5	49.89	104.8	87.30
85.7	52.15	106.1	88.44
87.0	54.4		

The following chart includes average weights for adult animals of various species.

Animal	Pounds	Kilograms
alpaca-male	132-176	60-80
-female	121	55
cat	6-10	3-5
chicken	4-6	2-3
dog-small	10-20	5-10
-medium	30-40	15-20
-large	60+	30+
duck	4-6	2-3
guanaco-male	220-330	100-150
-female	220-264	100-120
guinea pig	.8-1	.4-.5
llama-male	356-535	162-243
-female	238-415	108-189
rabbit	5-10	3-5
sheep	110-225	50-103
vicuna-male	88-143	40-65
-female	66-88	30-40

Horses

The following chart to determine weight after determining heart girth in cm.

Heart Girth (cm)	Pounds	Kilograms	Heart Girth (cm)	Pounds	Kilograms
69	82	37	103	208	94
73	84	38	105	221	100
77	91	41	107	234	106
79.5	96	44	109	247	112
81.5	103	47	111	259	118
85	114	52	113	273	124
87	122	55	115	287	130
89	131	60	117	302	137
91	141	64	119	316	144
93	152	69	121	331	150
95	163	74	123	347	158
97	173	79	125	362	164
99	185	84	127	377	171
101	196	89	129	393	179

Heart Girth (cm)	Pounds	Kilograms	Heart Girth (cm)	Pounds	Kilograms
131	409	186	169	788	358
133	425	193	171	812	369
135	441	200	173	836	380
137	459	209	175	861	391
139	477	217	177	888	404
141	496	225	179	916	416
143	515	234	181	945	430
145	532	242	183	974	443
147	553	251	185	1000	454
149	570	259	187	1030	468
151	588	267	189	1060	482
153	606	275	191	1087	494
155	628	285	193	1119	509
157	650	295	195	1148	522
159	673	306	197	1176	534
161	695	316	199	1206	548
163	718	326	201	1239	563
165	740	336	203	1272	578
167	765	348	205	1304	593

CALCULATING DOSAGES

Once an estimate or actual measure of the animal's weight has been determined, a dosage of medicine may be calculated. Calculations are made as follows:

animal's weight in kg X drug dose in mgs/kg = total number of mgs for that dose

Once the number of milligrams for the animal is determined, the amount of medicine can be determined. On the bottle of injectable medicine, the STRENGTH or CONCENTRATION will be listed in mg/ml. To enter the strength in this formula, turn the strength from the bottle upside down. For example, a bottle of oxytetracycline has a strength of 100 mg/ml. To put the strength into the formula, it is entered as 1 ml/100 mg.

total number of mgs for that dose X strength in ml/mg = number of mls for that dose

If the medicine is a tablet or bolus, the number of tablets or boluses may be determined using a similar formula.

$$\frac{\text{total number of mgs for that dose}}{\text{number of mgs in 1 tablet}} = \text{number of tablets for that dose}$$

Example 1

A 500 kilogram cow has pneumonia and needs to be treated with long-acting oxytetracycline with a strength of 200 mgs/ml.

First the number of milligrams should be determined. The dosage of long-acting oxytetracycline, as found in the formulary or on the bottle label, is 18 milligrams (mgs) per kilogram (kg) of body weight.

$$500\text{ kg} \times 18\text{ mg/kg} = 9000\text{ mg for that dose}$$

$$9000\text{ mg} \times \frac{1\text{ ml}}{200\text{ mg}} = 45\text{ ml of medicine for that dose}$$

Example 2

A 500 kg cow with pneumonia is to be treated with a long-acting sulfa bolus. The drug dose for sulfadimethoxine (Albon SR), as found in the formulary or on the label, is 137.5 mg/kg. Each tablet contains 12.5 grams.

$$500\text{ kgs} \times 137.5\text{ mg/kg} = 68{,}750\text{ mgs for that dose}$$

$$\frac{68{,}750\text{ mgs}}{12{,}500\text{ mgs}} = 5.5\text{ boluses}$$

Some medicines have the concentration given in international units (I.U./ml). The same steps for calculating the dose apply. For example, a 400 kg horse has a deep puncture wound so that it needs to be treated with penicillin having a strength of 300,000 I.U./ml. The dosage of procaine penicillin G, as found in the formulary, is 20,000 to 50,000 I.U./kg. The higher dosage found in the formulary is the dosage that is chosen.

$$400\text{ kg} \times 50{,}000\text{ I.U./kg} = 20{,}000{,}000\text{ I.U. for that dose}$$

Again, the strength found on the bottle is turned upside down when entered in the formula.

$$20{,}000{,}000\text{ I.U.} \times \frac{1\text{ ml}}{300{,}000\text{ I.U.}} = 66.6\text{ ml. for that dose}$$

When the dose for a large amount of medication comes out to be a fraction of an ml, the amount is rounded up to the nearest ml. The horse in this example would be given 67 ml of penicillin.

SECTION 4

MONITORING THE PATIENT

MONITORING THE PATIENT

PATIENT INFORMATION

An animal caretaker's job begins with gathering information about an individual animal or a particular herd or flock. Knowing the **NORMAL HABITS** of an animal or a group of animals is very important because behavior different from what is normal often indicates disease. If there is a change in behavior, appetite, or feces, then a history and a hands-on physical examination are needed.

The **HISTORY** of the animal includes the animal's age, breed, diet, sex (gender), where it came from, and other information that helps lead to the diagnosis.

In the hands-on **PHYSICAL EXAMINATION**, the animal's **TEMPERATURE**, **PULSE** (how fast the heart is beating), **RESPIRATION** (what the animal's breathing is like and how fast it is breathing), and **GUT SOUNDS** (sounds made as the gut works to digest food) are determined. A routine for doing the physical exam needs to be followed so that no part of the animal is overlooked. The routine may be to start at the tip of the nose and work back or to look at body systems. Doing the same routine each time makes it less likely that any part will be overlooked. The purpose of the exam is to reach a diagnosis. Once a diagnosis has been made, treatment should be started. Early treatment and careful monitoring of the animal to see that it is improving makes a good outcome more likely. If after 2-3 days the initial treatment is not working, the animal should be re-evaluated and treatment changed if necessary.

Some drugs may cause side effects in the animal or the animal may react to a drug in an unusual way. Treatment may need to be changed because of these reactions.

To follow are sections explaining history taking, physical examination, monitoring the patient, and side effects.

HISTORY (BACKGROUND)

The history is the background information on an animal. What has been happening to the animal helps the animal caretaker determine why the animal is now sick and what the cause of the sickness is likely to be. Questions that should be asked when taking a history include the following:

- How old is the animal?
- What breed is the animal?
- Is the animal male or female or neutered ?

- If female, is the animal pregnant? Has the animal birthed recently? Is the animal lactating?
- Is the animal new to the flock/herd?
- What, if any, vaccinations has the animal received and when?
- Has the animal traveled recently? If yes, where?
- How long has the animal been sick?
- Is there a possibility that the animal was injured?
- Has the animal received any medications?
- Has there been a change in feed or water?
- What feeds are being fed? How long have they been fed?
- Is the feed moldy or dusty?
- Is the feed the correct feed for the animal?
- Is the feed being given in adequate amounts for the animal?
- Are there any other animals involved?
- What was the first sign of illness noted?
- Have the signs changed?

Other questions may apply in a particular situation.

Physical Examination

The First Step: Watching the animal from a distance

Normal animals should be observed at least once a day to see if eating, drinking, feces, and general behavior are normal. Early signs of a problem may be only a slight change in appetite, less activity, a little more work to breathe, or feces that are too fluid or too firm. If the caretaker is not familiar with normal for that animal, these early changes could go unnoticed. Generally, the earlier an illness is detected and treatment begun, the more likely a successful outcome will result.

The animal is watched from a distance first because it may try to hide feeling ill if a person is close enough to be a threat. Birds will especially try to hide an illness. In the wild a sick animal hides the illness to protect itself from being singled out as an easy meal for a predator. Tame animals are less likely to try to look healthy as a person approaches. Also, something may be noticed from a distance that would be missed if the animal is close, such as the way it is standing or how it is holding its head.

A table and diagrams follow comparing normal animal behavior to behavior that is not normal (abnormal behavior).

Normal (fig. 4.1)

1. head- held up, looks alert
2. ears- held erect if it can hold them erect
3. nose- little to no clear discharge
4. walking- picking up feet as usual; not limping
5. posture- normal
6. feces and urine- normal in amount and appearance
7. grooming- usual grooming activity
8. chewing movements- normal when eating, not grinding teeth (chewing with no food or cud in the mouth)
9. belly-not kicking at belly, not stretching nor looking at stomach (signs of belly pain)
10. body in general- no swollen or bright red areas

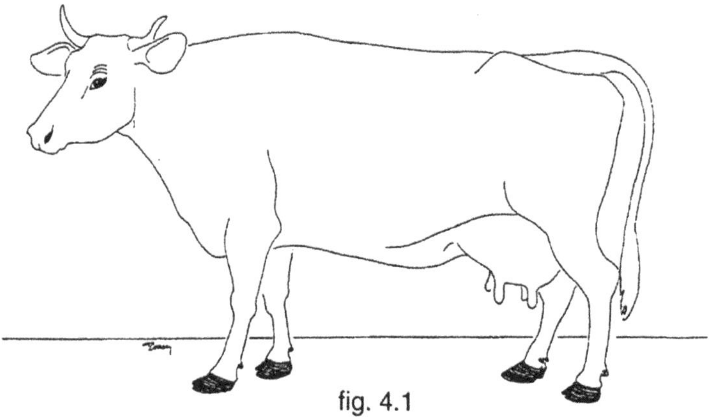

fig. 4.1

Abnormal (fig. 4.2)

1. head- hanging, looks dull or sleepy
2. ears- drooping
3. nose- cloudy discharge or a large amount of clear liquid present
4. walking- slower, possibly dragging feet, stiff or limping
5. posture- unusual, such as arched back or outstretched neck
6. feces and urine- straining to urinate or pass feces, increased or decreased frequency of passing urine or feces, urine or feces with blood, feces that are too fluid or too firm
7. grooming- hair coat or feathers rough, animal not grooming
8. chewing movements- grinding teeth, chewing when no food or cud is present
9. belly- kicking at belly, belly muscles tight with pain, bloated
10. body in general- swollen area, bright red area where it should not be bright red

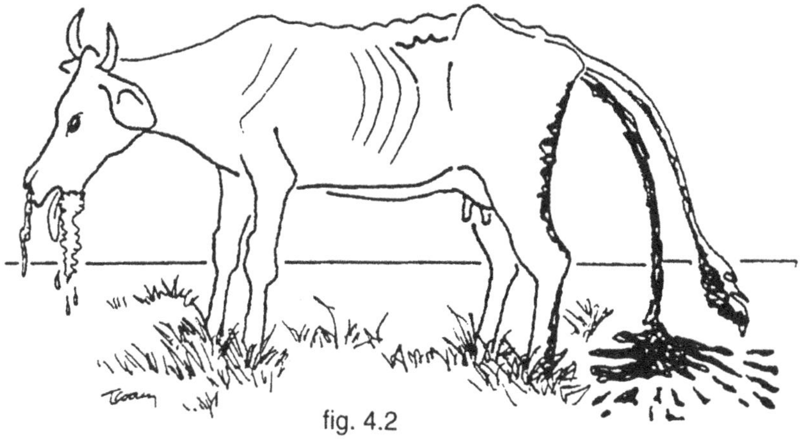

fig. 4.2

When an animal shows any of the signs noted under abnormal, the animal should be caught and given a hands-on physical exam to see why the sign or signs are present. It is better to do a physical exam where one may not have been necessary than to miss early treatment of a disease and lose an animal as the result.

HANDS-ON PHYSICAL EXAMINATION

In the hands-on physical exam to arrive at a diagnosis of an illness, the temperature, pulse, breathing, consistency of feces, and, depending on the species, activity of the gut are determined . Having a set routine when looking at an animal prevents overlooking a problem. Any problem may be a clue to what disease the animal has and clues help!

One possible routine is to start at the animal's head and work towards its tail. On the head, the eyes are checked for discharge, redness, and for cloudiness of the outer surface (cornea) or the inside (lens). The nose should be clean with a small amount of clear thin liquid present. More detail on the nose follows in the respiration section. The nostrils should not be flaring when breathing at rest. Flaring indicates that too much effort is being required to breathe. The ears should be upright or in a position usual for that animal. Holding the head to one side may indicate something is in the ear on that side or that the ear hurts because of an infection. Redness inside the ear may indicate an infection as well. Next, the mouth could be examined, checking for problems with the teeth, the tongue, the opening to the windpipe, and the glands around the mouth. The mouth is also a good place to look at the **MUCOUS MEMBRANES**. The mucous membranes normally are light pink and, when pressed with a finger, should turn white, but become pink again within 2 seconds. If it takes longer than 2 seconds to become pink or if the membranes are dark red or gray, the animal is having problems with circulating its blood because of too little fluid or toxins from a disease. While examining the mouth the breath should be smelled. A foul odor may indicate a problem with a tooth; a sweet odor of acetone indicates ketosis. The examiner needs to use all senses in the examination. Before leaving the head, it should be checked that no areas are swollen. The two sides of the head should look alike.

On the neck, both sides of the neck should look alike. Lymph nodes, located just to the front and above the shoulder blade, should not be noticeable. If swollen, an infection in the neck area may be the cause. The animal should be willing to move its head up and down and left and right. If the animal doesn't want to move its neck, either the muscles or the bones in the neck may be damaged.

The chest and belly of the animal can be examined for symmetry (both sides look the same). The chest is a good place to check for body score. Body score is seeing that the animal has the correct amount of muscle and fat present. In a normal animal the ribs should be only slightly visible under the skin. An animal at the right weight is given a body score of 5. If the ribs are obvious, the animal is too thin. The body score would be less than 5, down to 1 if the animal is really skinny, the backbone and hips stick out, and the animal is weak from too little food. The belly should follow in a smooth line from the chest. If the ribs are obvious and the belly sticks out, the animal may have fluid build up in the belly and may need deworming or may have a plugged up gut and need a laxative. While examining the chest and belly, the pulse, respiration, and gut sounds can be checked.

Body Condition Score

Scores range from 1 (thin, the point of being weak from too little food, skin stretched taut over the bones) to 9 (extremely fat, deposits of fat over ribs so that it is hard to feel the ribs, fat deposits on each side of the tail). Detail on scores 4, 5, and 6 will follow:

<u>Score 4</u>

- foreribs are not readily seen
- last 2 sets of ribs are seen
- backbone cannot be seen but can be felt with slight pressure
- backbone feels rounded rather than sharp
- full but straight muscling in the hindquarters

Score 5
- no ribs can be readily seen
- backbone can only be felt with firm pressure
- areas on the sides of the tail are filled but not mounded

Score 6
- ribs are fully covered
- hindquarters are plump and full
- noticeable sponginess over the foreribs and on each side of the tail
- extremely firm pressure required to feel backbone

At the tail end the temperature is taken. Details on temperature follow. On a female, the opening leading to the bladder and the uterus is located below the anus. It should be examined for discharge. If none is present on the opening, it may be present on the legs or tail. All three places are normally clean. The tail should also have hair present. If the anus is itching or irritated, hair may be rubbed off the backside of the tail. In a male animal, the testicles should both be the same size, firm but not hard, should have no hard areas in them, and should not be tender to light squeezing. The sheath should not be swollen and the male should be able to move the penis in and out without difficulty.

Finally, the legs are examined. The legs should not be swollen and should look similar to each other. If the problem is lameness, a detailed examination of the feet and legs is included. In the lameness examination, the first problem is to decide which leg is causing the lameness. If the animal will not put any weight on the sore leg, it is easy to decide which leg hurts. The reasons for an animal to feel enough pain to refuse to use a leg are most commonly a fracture, an abscess, or a stone, nail, or other foreign body stuck in the foot. If the lameness isn't so obvious, watching a four-legged animal as it trots makes it easier to pick out the sore leg because at the trot only two legs are on the ground at a time. Since there are only two legs on the ground, each leg has to support half the animal's weight. The increased weight causes more pain, making the lameness more obvious.

Once the leg causing the pain is determined, that leg is thoroughly examined. Lameness is most commonly caused by a problem in the foot. The leg should be picked up, the foot thoroughly cleaned, and checked for a foreign body (nail, thorn, stone), a change in color from a bruise or an abscess, and checked for a wound. An abscess would have to be opened and cleaned. A foreign body would have to be removed and the area cleaned. A wound would require cleaning and possibly stitches. Antibiotics should be used. If nothing can be seen, a tool called a hoof tester can be used to put pressure on specific areas of the foot to see if the animal flinches. Any spot where the animal flinches should be examined more closely.

If no problem can be found in the foot, the leg should be examined. Looking at the leg for swelling or a change in shape can uncover a fracture or abscess. Feeling the leg for less obvious swelling or heat can uncover the same things or a sprain of tendons or the ligaments. Squeezing an area in question should make the animal flinch. Treatment based on the findings should be pursued. Rest may be the only treatment needed.

Temperature

All warm blooded animals maintain the body at a particular temperature that lets the body work at its best. Changes in that temperature, either an increase (fever) or a decrease (hypothermia), indicate a problem.

The temperature is taken using a rectal thermometer (fig. 4.3). The animal should be restrained so that it won't break the thermometer by moving or struggling. The thermometer should be held by the person taking the temperature or a long string should be attached to the thermometer since action of the muscles of the animal's rectum can move the thermometer up into the animal and out of reach or expel and break it. In larger animals the bulb of the thermometer should be held against the lining of the rectum. If allowed to sit in the middle of the rectum, the temperature may be mistakenly low.

The thermometer must be shaken down by holding the ring end firmly and using a snapping motion of the wrist. This motion moves the mercury in the thermometer below the lowest temperature expected. The thermometer should be held in the animal for 1 minute. The temperature is read by turning the thermometer until the mercury column appears wide. The number the column of mercury reaches is the animal's temperature (Fig. 4.3).

If a thermometer breaks, the silver liquid that comes out is mercury. Mercury is extremely toxic and should not be handled. Using gloves and paper to scoop up the tiny balls it forms and putting it in the sharps container or other container for material labeled **"BIOHAZARD"** would be the best way to dispose of it.

Normal temperature values for various species are recorded in the chart that follows.

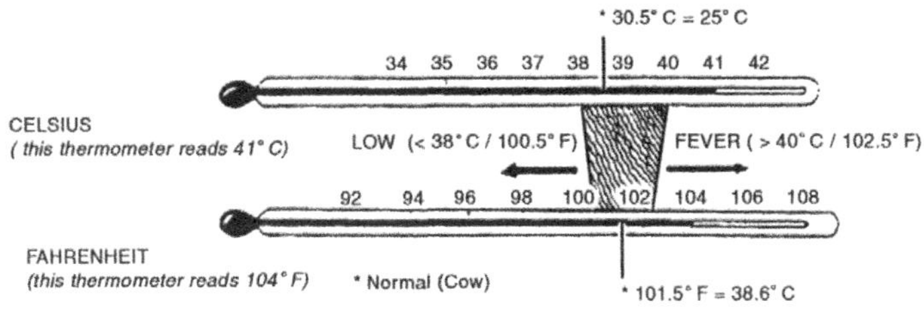

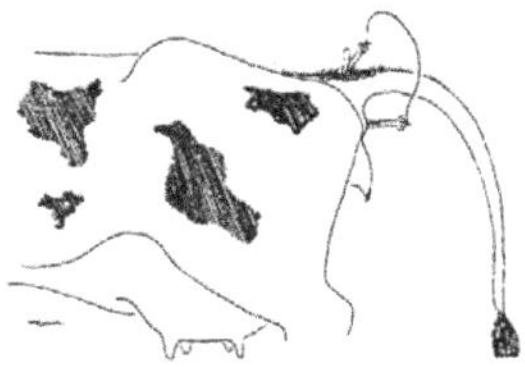

fig. 4.3

Pulse

Each animal has a heart rate. This pumping by the heart pushes blood (oxygen and food) to all parts of the body and takes wastes away from all parts of the body with the best timing for that animal. Generally, the smaller the animal the faster the heart rate.

The pulse of the animal may be taken by feeling the heart beat (fig. 4.4). This is done by resting a hand on the animal's ribs, on the left side, just behind the front leg. If a stethoscope is available, listening in the same spot will give the heart rate. Beats are counted for one minute. Pulse may also be determined by feeling a large artery. In horses and cattle, feeling the artery just under the angle of the jaw will give a pulse. In smaller animals (sheep, goats, dogs, cats) the pulse may be felt in the artery inside the back leg (see diagrams). Normal values for pulse, in beats per minute, are in the chart to follow.

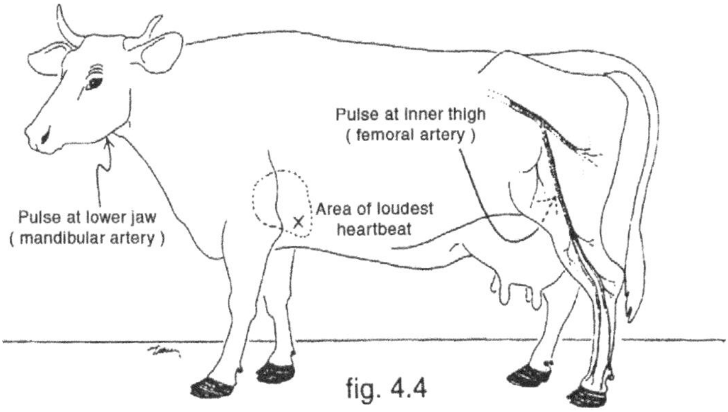

fig. 4.4

Respiration

As with the heart rate, the respiratory rate (how fast the animal is breathing) depends on how much oxygen the animal is using. After exercise, both the heart rate and the respiratory rate will be increased. With an infection in the lungs or when an animal has a fever, the respiratory rate will increase.

Respiratory rate is determined by counting the rise and fall (rise plus fall is one breath) of the ribs for 1 minute. How the animal is breathing is also important. If the animal is having trouble getting breath, it should be watched to see if the animal is having more trouble when inhaling (breathing in) or when exhaling (breathing out). If the trouble is when inhaling, the difficulty is probably in the part of the animal's airway from the nose to the windpipe. If the trouble is when exhaling, the difficulty is more likely in the lungs, such as pneumonia. If material is coming from the nose, it should be examined. Large amounts of a clear, thin liquid indicates a viral infection. A cloudy discharge that is thick and gray to yellow indicates a bacterial infection. Blood in small amounts may be seen in infections. Large amounts of blood generally indicate a serious problem. Normal respiratory rates are recorded in the chart to follow.

Gut Sounds

In ruminants (cattle, sheep, goats) the rumen should have 2-4 contractions per minute. This compartment of the stomach is used as a fermentation and mixing vat. The rumen is best heard by listening with a stethoscope just behind the ribs on the animal's left side (fig. 4.5). The contraction may also be felt by placing a hand firmly on the animal's left side just behind the ribs. The contraction (muscles of the gut moving) is heard as a gurgling, scratching noise, starting quietly, getting louder, then getting quieter again. The side of the animal may bulge out when the sound is the loudest. More or fewer contractions per minute indicates a problem.

Horses produce gut sounds that can be heard with a stethoscope in the flank area, between the ribs and the hip. Listening close to the back, then close to the belly on both sides for 1 minute at each spot gives an idea of how the gut is working. A chart (see drawing) may be used to keep track of the movement and gas sounds in the gut. Normally, 2-4 contractions should be heard in each spot during 1 minute of listening. Tinkling sounds of gas bubbling through the fluid in the gut should only be heard 2-4 times per minute as well. More or fewer contractions or more gas sounds can all be a source of pain in the horse's belly, that belly pain being referred to as colic. Normal numbers of gut sounds are recorded in the chart to follow:

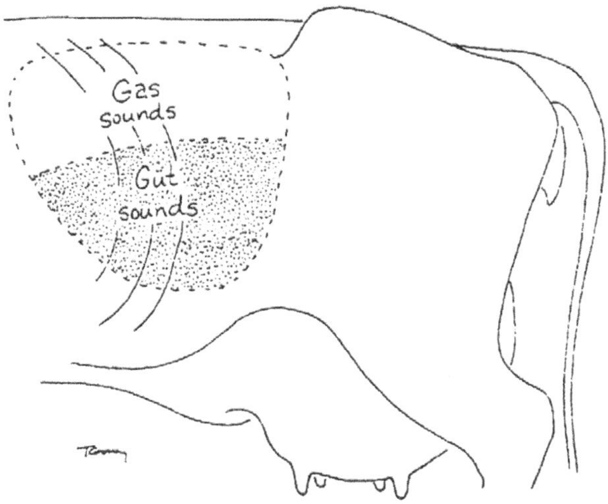

fig. 4.5

ANIMAL	TEMPERATURE*	PULSE**	RESPIRATION***	GUT SOUNDS****
horse	99.5-100.4(37.5-38.5)	30-40	9-10	2-4
pig	100.4-104.0(38-40)	63-92	10-20	N/A
cattle	99.5-102.5(37.5-39.2)	70-90	12-16	2-4
sheep	101.3-104.4(38.5-40.0)	70-80	12-15	2-4
goat	101.3-104.9(38.5-40.5)	70-80	12-15	2-4
llama	99.0-101.8(37.2-38.7)	60-90	10-30	2-4
camel	97.5-107.6(36.4-42)	40-50	5-12	?
rabbit	100.4-104.0(38-39.6)	130-325	32-60	N/A
guinea pig	100.0-103.1(37.8-39.5)	260-400	100-150	N/A
dog	99.5-102.2(37.5-39)	60-120	14-20	N/A
cat	100.4-103.1(38-39.5)	100-140	20-30	N/A
poultry	104.9-109.4(40.5-43)	180-440	15-30	N/A

*Temperature is in degrees Fahrenheit and (degrees Centigrade).
**Pulse is in beats per minute.
***Respiration is in breaths (breathe in plus breathe out is one breath)per minute.
****Gut sounds is in contractions (muscles of the gut moving) per minute.

Younger animals (less than 1 year) may have a pulse and respiratory rate up to twice the lower value listed. Their temperature may be 1-2 degrees higher than the upper value listed for the adult. In animals where a range of sizes may be seen, as with dogs, smaller dogs will have the higher values and larger dogs will have the lower values.

PATIENT MONITORING

Keeping track of an animal's response to treatment is important in deciding if the treatment is working. It would be best if an animal is examined twice daily. If the patient is getting better, the course of medication should be continued at least 2 days after signs of illness have disappeared. If the patient's condition is worsening or if there is no change after 2-3 days, the diagnosis should be reevaluated and treatment changed if necessary.

Good written records help. Trying to remember pulse, temperature or respiration for several hours, let alone from day to day, is difficult. Written records also are something that can be reexamined later.

Keeping good records makes the decision process of whether the treatment is working or needs to be changed easier. A form follows which may assist in keeping track of treatment information.

Form

This form can be copied and used to keep track of the daily exams of an animal being treated. An explanation of each entry to be made follows.

Explanation of Terms

Diagnosis - The diagnosis is the name of the animal's disease. If the disease isn't known, the main problem, for example "bloody diarrhea", may be used. Final diagnosis may be the same as the initial diagnosis or may have changed as new clinical signs appeared.

Patient Identification (ID) - The animal being treated needs to be specifically identified with a numbered ear tag, a paint stick or some other means that will last as long as the animal is being treated. Permanent identification would be the best. Sick animals should be in a different location than healthy animals, but if this is not possible, the ID mark ensures the correct animal is being treated.

Animal Caretaker - It is important for one person to be responsible for the care of an animal. Treatment might be neglected if two people each think the other is attending to the animal. Also, double treatment should not take place by two people who each think they are responsible.

Date - Spaces in the date category may be used to record morning and evening information, or day by day.

Temperature, pulse, respiration, gut sounds, urine, and feces - These values should be recorded in the appropriate spot. Amount and appearance of urine and feces should be recorded. Knowing these volumes will help determine if the amount of fluid the animal is drinking is keeping up with the amount it is losing.

Attitude - Attitude is an extremely important indicator of how the animal feels. Is the animal alert? Depressed? Conscious? Unconscious? Active? Reluctant to move? These are the types of signs to observe and record for the attitude.

Fluid Intake - This area of the sheet is for recording the amount of fluid going into the animal. Keeping track of how much fluid is entering the animal is very important whenever dehydration is a concern. The amount of fluid going in must match the amount leaving the animal, especially when diarrhea or excessive urine production is part of the problem. Fever, sweating, or an increased respiratory rate will increase fluid loss as well.

Route - Route means how the fluid is entering the animal's body. If the animal is drinking, the route is called oral or PO. If the fluid is given into a vein through a needle, the route is called IV. If the fluids are given under the skin, to be absorbed by the animal's blood system, that route is called subcutaneous or SQ. (This route is usually used only in smaller animals because of the limited volume that may be given by the SQ route.)

Type - Type of fluid that will best help the animal differs with the route and the animal's needs. With loss of fluid through diarrhea, various salts added to the water help the water get into the body and correct losses of these salts that are necessary for normal body function. For intravenous (IV) fluids, the fluid must be sterile. Lactated Ringer's solution (LRS) has many salts in it and is given IV. If extra energy is needed, glucose may be added to the solution. Normal saline (NS or 0.9% NaCl) may also be given in certain situations. Record what type of fluid is being given. The solutions given IV may also be given under the skin (subcutaneously or SQ).

Feed - The type of food and the amount of food being eaten are excellent indicators of how the animal is feeling.

Medications - The remainder of the monitoring sheet is for recording the type of drug, amount given, how the medication is given (oral, injected), and how often it is given..

INITIAL DIAGNOSIS ______________ FINAL DIAGNOSIS ______________

PATENT ID______________ ANIMAL CARETAKER ______________

DATE					
TEMPERATURE					
PULSE					
RESPIRATION					
GUT SOUNDS					
URINE					
STOOL					
ATTITUDE					
FLUID INTAKE ROUTE					
TYPE					
FEED					
MEDICATIONS ANTIBIOTICS					
ANTIINFLAM.					
OTHER					

SIDE EFFECTS

A side effect occurs when a drug works in the animal's body in a way that is not normal. Some animals experience side effects more often than others. Cats, for example, tend to be more sensitive to the effects of drugs than other animals. An individual animal may be more sensitive to a particular drug than other animals of the same kind. The side effects may be mild enough that the drug can still be used or it may have to be stopped and a different drug used.

An allergic reaction is one type of side effect. The animal's immune system, the system of the body that protects it from diseases or tissues that are not its own, is responding to the drug as if it were a threat to the body. The response of the body causes the signs. An allergic reaction may be immediate or delayed (happening several hours or days later). The immediate reaction is the most life threatening and is most often seen when giving vaccinations. The animal may stagger, have problems breathing, become weak, fall down or show muscle spasms. **IMMEDIATE TREATMENT WITH EPINEPHRINE IS REQUIRED TO SAVE THE ANIMAL'S LIFE**. If a drug other than a vaccine has caused the reaction, treatment with that drug should be stopped. Antihistamines, corticosteroids and nonsteroidal anti-inflammatories may also help the animal to recover.

A delayed reaction occurs after the animal has been receiving a medication for a time OR it occurs hours after the medication was given. Swellings in the skin, swellings around the eyes, and itchiness are typical signs. Stopping use of the drug and use of antihistamines, corticosteroids and nonsteroidal anti-inflammatories help recovery. Antibiotics, vaccines and insecticides can cause a delayed reaction.

When too much of a particular drug is given, an animal has received an **OVERDOSE**. If the drug was given by injection, the drug cannot be removed from the animal. Careful reading of the drug package insert will give information on what signs to watch for and how to treat the overdose. Many times just keeping the animal quiet, warm, and in a place where it cannot injure itself is all that can be done.

If an overdose of an oral drug has been given and the drug is not extremely damaging to skin and membranes, the animal may be made to vomit. Dogs and cats may be made to vomit by giving hydrogen peroxide (10 to 30 cc) or salt (a teaspoon of table salt in the back of the throat). In animals that don't vomit, such as cattle, horses, sheep, goats, llamas, and camels, mineral oil (a pint to a gallon, depending on size of the animal), activated charcoal (one to two cups, depending on the size of the animal, stirred into water), and Epsom salts (several tablespoons to two cups, depending on the size of the animal, dissolved in water), in combination or individually may be given. Giving these can prevent the drug from entering the body or push it through the gut quickly thereby decreasing how much gets into the body. Generally, use the Epsom salts and activated charcoal if the substance overdosed is oily and use the mineral oil and activated charcoal if the substance is not oily.

When a drug that is used topically has been overdosed, washing the animal will remove the drug and stop any more drug from entering the body. Remember to check the package insert for specific information on a specific drug.

SECTION **5**

THE MEDICINE CABINET

THE MEDICINE CABINET

DEFINITIONS

Hygiene - cleanliness

Disinfection - the destruction (death) of most living microorganisms. Disinfection does not kill bacterial spores (some bacteria have this protective shell), tubercle bacteria (tuberculosis), or some viruses unless it says so on the label. These must be killed by sterilization.

Disinfectant - a chemical agent that destroys (kills) disease-producing bacteria and viruses. Disinfectants cannot be used on skin.

Antiseptics - chemical agents that destroy most organisms and can be used on skin

Sterilization - the complete destruction of living organisms

HYGIENE OF THE VETERINARY TECHNICIAN AND THE ANIMAL PATIENT

The veterinary technician has two goals to prevent spreading disease -- protecting himself and protecting the patient. If the animal is suspected of having a disease which could infect the veterinary technician, then precautions such as gloves or plastic sleeves, mask, rubber apron, or coveralls must be worn. If in doubt, then it is better to be protected.

To protect the animal the veterinary technician must be CLEAN. Wash your hands with soap both before and after treating a patient. Clothing contaminated from handling a sick animal should be changed or covered before examining new animals. All tools or instruments must be cleaned and disinfected or sterilized. Needles and syringes must be sterile. Wipe the rubber top of an injectable medicine bottle with disinfectant prior to inserting the needle. Germs are transmitted primarily through touching -- by you! by your tools! by sick animals! BE CLEAN!

Injection sites must be free of dirt and wiped with an antiseptic prior to inserting the needle. If not, dirt and microorganisms will be carried into the animal on the needle and cause an infection. Dirt, body fluids, pus and dead tissue debris should be washed away prior to applying topical medicines. An animal's mouth should be free of feed or grass when giving oral medicine so that it will be swallowed without difficulty.

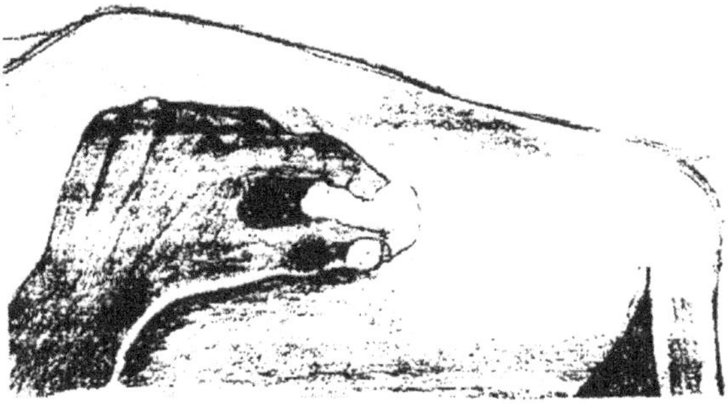

DISINFECTION AND STERILIZATION OF VETERINARY INSTRUMENTS

PURPOSE: Keep the instruments which are to be used on animals in good working order, cleaned and disinfected (or sterile) in order to do a good job and prevent the spread of disease.

STEPS:

1) Clean instruments well with soap and water. Dirt, blood and dried fluids must be removed by careful washing. Rinse well with clean water.
2) Disinfect or sterilize.

Disinfection. Place the instruments in a chemical agent for the period of time recommended by the label directions. Disinfection time is influenced by the type of material being disinfected, the amount of dirt and germs, the strength (concentration) of the disinfectant and its germ-killing ability. ADVANTAGES: disinfection does not dull instruments; easy; economical. DISADVANTAGES: many disinfectants irritate tissues so rinse instruments well with sterile water; ineffective against bacterial spores, tubercle bacteria and many viruses.

Sterilization. There are many methods: boiling, dry heat, steam under pressure, and chemical agents (gases or liquids). Each method has advantages and disadvantages.

1. Dry heat (oven). Glassware and metal items without sharp edges should be held at 170 C for l hour. Powders, oils, waxes, and petrolatum products should be placed in 30 ml units and held at 160 C for 2 hours. Sharp instruments should be held at a temperature of 150 C for 3 hours.[22] ADVANTAGES: best method to sterilize oils, powders, petroleum products, needles and sharp instruments; needles and sharp instruments are less likely to rust. DISADVANTAGES: heat can be difficult to control;

destroys fabrics and rubber items; may destroy the temper (hardness) of metal instruments; the process requires a slow rise and fall of the heat.

2. Boiling. Method: Bring water to a rapid boil. Add instruments and allow to boil for 30 minutes. ADV: inexpensive. DISADV: will not destroy spore-forming organisms unless an alkali agent is added (such as sodium carbonate 2% or sodium hydroxide 1%.[22] These alkalis should not be used when boiling glassware or rubber items.); can rust instruments; dulls sharp instruments.
3. Saturated steam under pressure. Sterilization with this method is accomplished in a pressure cooker or in a machine called an autoclave. Only materials that are not damaged by either heat or moisture and are penetrable by steam are effectively sterilized. Proper placement of instruments and instrument packs within the autoclave must be done to get adequate steam flow around them. In gravity displacement sterilizers at 121 C sterilization times range from 13 minutes for small items to 30 minutes for large packs. In prevacuum sterilizers at 131 C even large packs can be sterilized in 4 minutes.[22] ADV: penetrates well; economical. DISADV: dulls sharp instruments; scorches fabrics; will wet contents if operated improperly; will not sterilize through grease, oils, or proteins; damages some instruments and supplies (especially plastic and rubber).

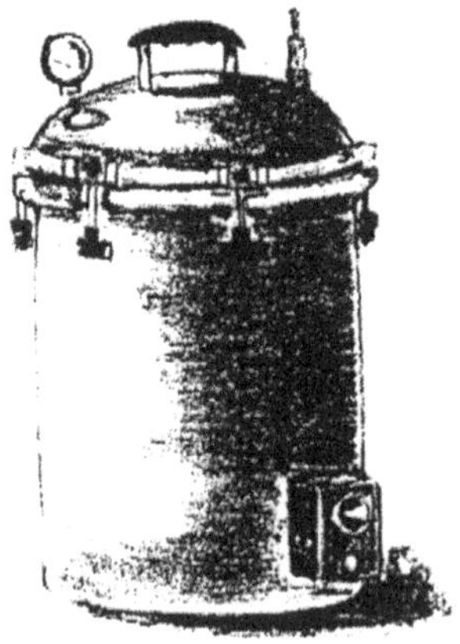

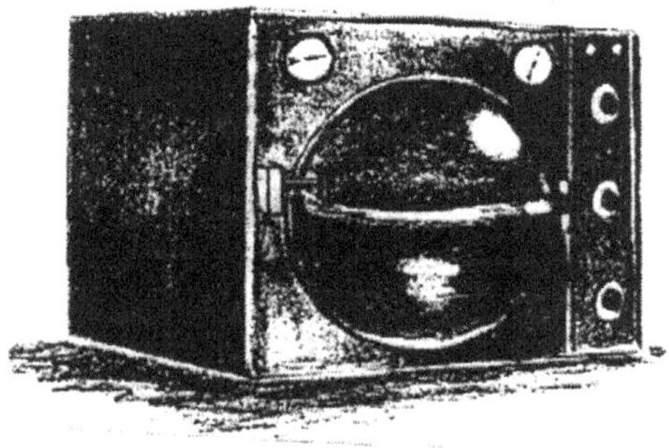

4. Chemicals. Chemicals used for sterilization are the same as disinfectants (kill disease producing bacteria and viruses) plus they kill spores, viruses, and tubercle bacteria. Sterilization time varies from 3 to 24 hours. 2% alkalinized aqueous glutaraldehyde solution is an example of a chemical sterilization agent.

REUSE OF INSTRUMENTS

Most instruments used in the treatment of animals can be reused. Common sense often will determine when an instrument no longer works properly or cannot be cleaned or sterilized adequately. At this point the instrument must be disposed of properly or repaired.

Syringes. Both glass and plastic syringes can be cleaned, sterilized and reused. The number of times this can be done varies with the type of syringe.

Needles. Needles must be sharp so as little damage as possible is done to the animal. Needles come in two varieties: 1) disposable and 2) reusable stainless steel. Both types can be reused although disposable needles will get dull and bend easily. All needles can be sharpened with a whetstone prior to sterilization. Needles can become obstructed with dried blood, pus, body fluids, or thick medicines. Rinsing with clean water immediately after use will help prevent clogging of needles. A fine wire or smaller needle can be used to clean out a clogged needle although some residue may remain. REMEMBER even the smallest bit of blood or fluid can transmit a germ to another animal so BE CLEAN AND STERILE!

HANDLING, STORAGE AND SECURITY OF DRUGS AND INSTRUMENTS

Manufacturers give specific instructions concerning the use, handling, and storage of drugs. These instructions are on the label or in the instruction paper, called a package insert, that comes with the drug. ALWAYS read and follow those instructions! A veterinarian may provide additional information which may not be on the label.

DO NOT use a medicine without knowing exactly what it is. All drugs should be labeled. If the label is damaged and cannot be read easily then replace it with at least the name of the drug, strength (usually in mg/ml or mg), and expiration date. A piece of tape, a piece of paper or a tag with this information clearly written on it could be attached in some manner to the drug's container.

DO NOT use a drug beyond its expiration date. It may have lost its strength.

DO NOT use a medicine that has changed color, has particles in it, had a contaminated needle inserted into it, or has been changed in any way. Ask a veterinarian about the change and about the medicine's use.

DO protect glass instruments and medicine bottles against breakage in transport and use. Gently crumpled paper can be put around bottles to help prevent breaking when carried in a box, sack or pack. Place paper of cotton in containers partly filled with tablets or boluses prevent the tablets from breaking during transport.

DO NOT store medicines in direct sunlight or in places likely to be exposed to very hot or freezing temperatures. **ALL** vaccines should be refrigerated or stored on ice unless the label gives other instructions.

DO store powders and tablets in dry places. Dampness could damage them.

DO STORE ALL MEDICINES AND INSTRUMENTS IN A SAFE PLACE. Choose areas where children, animals, and thieves cannot get into easily. Putting them in a locked box or locked room is best. Placing them on high shelves should make it hard for children and most animals to reach.

DO make sure all medicine containers have tight fitting lids or

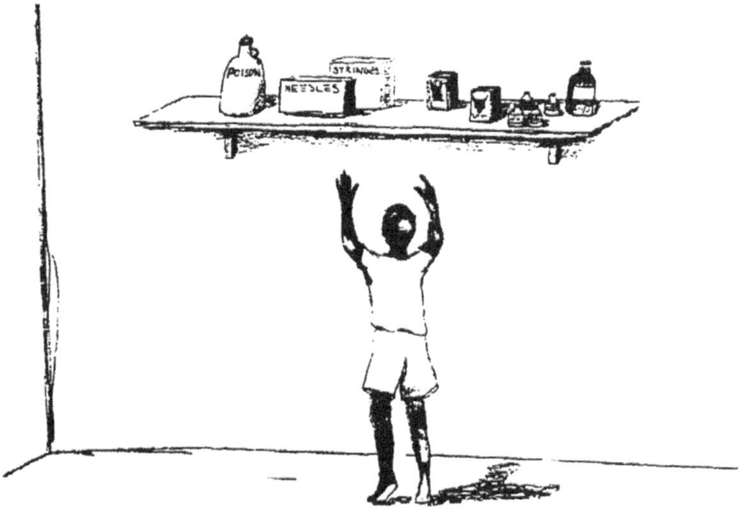

caps. This will keep out insects, moisture, and provide some security against children and animals.

DISPOSAL OF VETERINARY DRUGS AND INSTRUMENTS

Veterinarians and veterinary technicians must do their work in the most honest and ethical way. This includes getting rid (disposal) of all medicine and instruments when they are no longer needed. DO NOT throw these things on the ground for another person to pick up. It is your responsibility as an animal health provider to promote a good image of veterinary medicine. Proper disposal is part of this responsibility.

Read the label or package insert for any special instructions regarding disposal. Some medicines and vaccines need to be burned or sterilized before final disposal.

Sharp items, such as suture needles, injection needles and scalpel blades must be collected in thick plastic bottles (gallon bottles are ideal). These bottles are capped, sterilized and then taken to a human or veterinary hospital for final disposal. It may be permissible to fill the bottle with plaster of Paris, concrete, or mud to be buried after the mixture has dried. Ask an animal or human health care worker what should be done in your area.

Glass articles can be deeply buried (0.5 meter of dirt should cover them). This must be done in an area set aside by a health care worker for this purpose.

THE PACKAGE INSERT

-- This is the printed instruction page provided with all medication.

This information is provided by the manufacturer or producer of the drug. The content will be different for each medicine, but all the important information will be given. The information will be organized into sections, and these sections will be seen clearly because the section headings will be in darker print or enlarged lettering or both.

Explanation Of The Section Headings

Remember, not all these sections will be given in each package insert.

DRUG NAME -- The name given by the manufacturer ("trade name") is first, followed by the generic name. The generic name is the same for the same drug from ALL manufacturers.

SPECIES: This section lists the animals in which the drug can be used safely. This information often follows the name of the drug or is in the **DESCRIPTION** section.

NOTE: A veterinarian may give information about a drug's use in another type of animal. This is called "off-label" use. DO NOT use a medicine unless you are sure it is proper to do so!

DESCRIPTION: 1) general type of medicine -- such as antibiotic or hormone or disinfectant 2) brief explanation of what it does 3) chemical name and some chemical properties.

ACTION:

PHARMACOLOGY: This section tells the specific ways the drug works in the body. Without special training, this section can be difficult to understand.

RECOMMENDED USES:

INDICATIONS: This section tells the diseases for which the drug can be used and/or the specific germs for which the drug can be used.

DOSAGE AND ADMINISTRATION:

HOW TO APPLY: This section tells how much of the drug should be given in one dose and how often it should be given. For help in determining dosages see section 3. This section may also give limits on the use of the drug -- for example, the drug's use may be forbidden in young, growing animals.

CAUTIONS:

PRECAUTIONS:

SAFETY:

WARNING:

CONTRAINDICATIONS:

SIDE EFFECTS:

ADVERSE REACTIONS:

DRUG INTERACTIONS:

OVERDOSAGE:

ANIMAL TOXICOLOGY:

TOXICITY: These sections give advice about the drug's use, including very important information about the problems which MAY be seen when using the drug.

WITHDRAWAL: This section tells how long following treatment to avoid consumption of milk and/or meat of the treated animal. These instructions should be strictly followed to prevent people from getting sick from eating the meat or drinking the milk of a treated animal.

HOW SUPPLIED: This section tells the size of containers the drug comes in -- such as 1000 tablets or 100 ml vial, and the strengths (concentrations) of the drug -- such as
50 mg/ml and 250 mg/ml or 100 mg tablets and 200 mg tablets.

STORAGE CONDITIONS: how to store the medicine while it is not being used.

NOTE TO PHYSICIAN: This section tells a physician how to treat human exposure to the drug.

It would be prudent to keep the package inserts in a safe place, such as a filing cabinet or notebook, where they could be easily reached and read when needed.

DRUG CONTAINER LABELS which are attached by the manufacturer to the medicine container will have some of the above information. The information will be limited by the size of the container and will tell you to read the package insert for complete information.

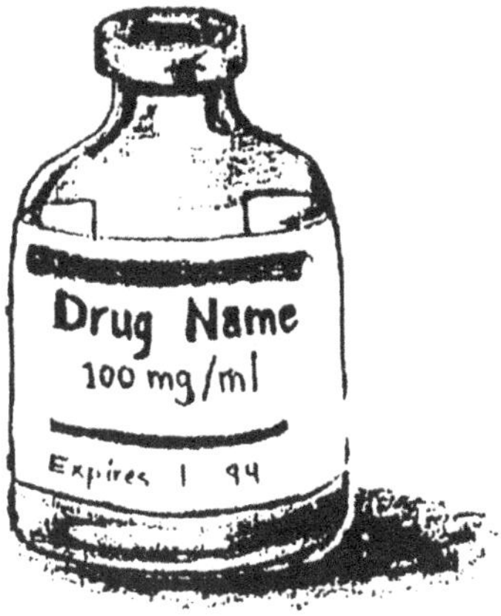

SECTION 6

METHODS OF DRUG ADMINISTRATION

METHODS OF DRUG ADMINISTRATION

DEFINITIONS

Absorption - the passing of a substance across a tissue and into the blood

Abscess - a pocket of pus

Aspirate - During the administration of an injection, the veterinary technician pulls back on the plunger of a syringe looking for fluid in the hub of the needle or the tip of the syringe. This technique is used to detect whether or not the needle is in a blood vessel. One can use this technique with an empty syringe and needle to detect or drain a seroma or abscess.

Euthanasia - to kill an animal with a humane method to prevent suffering

Gastrointestinal stasis - when movement of food out of the stomach and through the intestines has stopped

IM - intramuscular; in the muscle

IP - intraperitoneal; into the abdominal (coelomic) cavity

IV - intravenous; in the vein

Seroma - pocket of clear to reddish, watery body fluid

SQ or SC - subcutaneous; under the skin

CONSIDERATIONS OF MEDICATION

After performing an examination and making a diagnosis, BUT before administering any drugs or vaccines the veterinary technician must ask himself some very important questions. With experience these questions will be done without having to think about it, but in the beginning the technician may want to prepare a list so that none will be forgotten.

1. Can people or other animals catch the disease? If so, then take the needed precautions.
2. Is the animal well enough to take the medicine or vaccine? Many injectable drugs need to be given once or twice daily. Is the animal in good enough condition to take injections or will these make the animal hurt so that it will not want to eat and drink or walk? Some drugs cause an animal to feel bad as a normal side effect. Will this add to its illness so that it will give up and die? In some cases strengthening an animal with good nursing care prior to treatment or providing extra nursing care along with treatment is needed. Perhaps the best drug for a disease should not be used if the animal's problems will not allow it.

3. How much restraint is required to give the animal its medicine? Will the restraint likely harm or weaken it?
4. After the proper medicine is chosen, how should it be given? Various factors need to be considered. For example, if the animal is vomiting then oral medicines probably will be vomited out before having any effect. If diarrhea is a symptom then oral medicines may not be taken into the body properly and therefore they will not work. If there are large areas of raw, broken skin then a topical medicine may enter the body in large amounts and cause internal damage. One can change the way a drug is given if new symptoms develop or as symptoms disappear.
5. What are the normal side effects of the medicine? What is the WITHDRAWAL TIME for meat and milk? What are the toxic side effects? <u>The owner must be told about these things.</u>
6. If a medicine is to be dispensed to the sick animal's owner, can he or she give it at the right time and in the right manner?
7. When should improvement be seen? Will it be gradual or quick? What is the next thing to do if no improvement happens? Tell the owner what to expect and when you should be consulted again if needed. <u>Medicines are not guaranteed to work and this should be told to the owner.</u> Some diseases cannot be treated. Treatment may be a waste of time and money. Perhaps the animal should be slaughtered and eaten (IF IT SAFE TO DO SO) or perhaps it should be euthanized and disposed of properly. BE HONEST WITH THE OWNER -- this will keep their trust even if the treatment does not work.

MEDICATION TYPES

Medications (drugs) can be delivered to an animal in many ways:

1. <u>Injectable.</u> These drugs go IV, IM, SQ, or IP. Most drugs can be found in an injectable form, although they may not be readily available or affordable. This method of administering a drug is very important because it does not rely on an animal's digestive system, it is relatively simple to do, it is reliable, and it works quickly.
2. <u>Oral.</u> These drugs are given directly into the mouth or into the esophagus or stomach with a tube. Many drugs can be given this way. Oral medications are given as tablets, capsules, boluses, liquids, and powders. This method is often used because it is easy, effective, safe, and usually the least expensive.

3. Topical. These medications are put on top of the skin, eye, or wound. Some drug classes used this way are insecticides, antibiotic salves, eye salves and drops, and wound healing creams, powders and sprays. Areas treated with topicals include eyes, ears, open wounds, limbs, joints and skin.
4. Intramammary. These medications are put into the milk bag through the teat canal.

WHEN GIVING MEDICATIONS ALWAYS FOLLOW THE LABEL DIRECTIONS OR A VETERINARIAN'S INSTRUCTIONS.

Injections

Injections must be given in the proper manner to help avoid problems. The most common problem is pain. Pain is a result of the needle going into the skin and the stretching of the tissues by the medicine to make room for the medication. Also, certain drugs sting the tissues when they are injected. This pain cannot be eliminated but injecting the medication slowly will sometimes reduce this pain. If the animal moves after the needle is inserted, then it is possible for the needle to damage the tissues. Adequate restraint is very important to minimize this.

Injections must be given in the proper place to minimize the formation of an abscess or a seroma. Swelling can occur with a SQ or IM injection but usually will go down in 3-5 days. Warm to hot, moist compresses applied to the area 3 to 4 times per day may help heal these. If the swelling stays and the site softens, then an abscess or seroma has developed. Oftentimes abscesses grow and burst open to drain before they will heal. Opening up the skin into the abscess to make it drain will help it heal more quickly. If the abscess cannot open to the outside then it will drain inside the animal. In this situation the animal could take a very long time to heal. Abscesses or seromas develop as a result of (1) a dirty needle, (2) dirty skin, (3) too much medicine injected in the site, or (4) too small of a blood supply into the site where the medicine was injected. IM injections should be given into the middle of large muscles. SQ injections should be given under the skin and not in the skin.

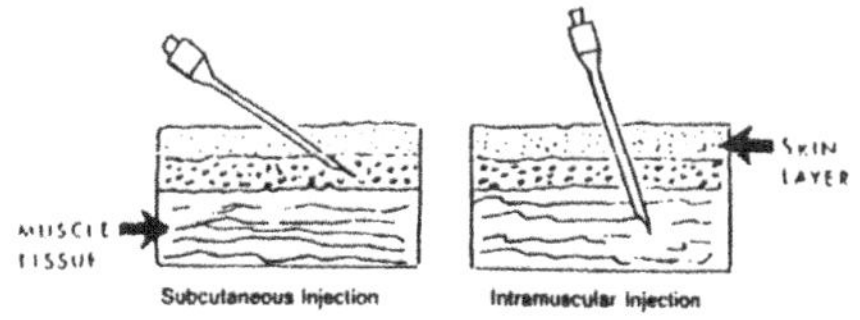

Proper needle placement for IV injection

Make sure the needle is in the vein for an IV injection by aspirating blood into the syringe prior to giving the injection. The usual site for the IV injection is the jugular vein. Behind this vein is an artery which contains blood at a higher pressure than the vein -- this blood is on its way to the head. Normal venous blood is a dark red and that from an artery is a bright red. IV injections should **ALWAYS** go in the vein. When medicine is injected into the artery, the animal will become immediately and seriously ill. The patient may stagger and fall down or seizure. A seizuring animal will be down on the ground with its legs moving as if it is running, or it will shake uncontrollably with its head and neck stretched towards its back. Some of these animals will die either from shock or from the seizure. Others will get back on their feet and return to normal within minutes or perhaps within days.

How to read and use a syringe

The veterinary agent should think of a syringe as both a tool that measures and one that administers a medicine. One could see it as a spoon or cup used for cooking in which flour is measured and then delivered to a bowl. A syringe measures the correct amount of a medicine and then is used to give the medicine to an animal. Syringes can be used for injecting or for giving medicines (without the needle) into the mouth to be swallowed.

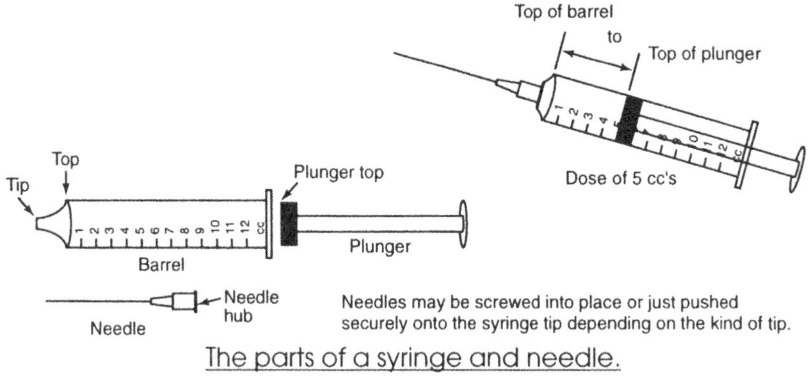

The parts of a syringe and needle.

All syringes have the same parts. The volume or amount of medicine is measured from the top of the plunger to the tip of the syringe. Each syringe must have a volume scale in "cc" on the barrel so that precise amounts can be measured. Most drugs require precise dosing to (1) prevent serious side effects, (2) to work the best in the animal, and (3) to prevent waste. If the scale is not readable then the syringe should not be used to measure medicines for an animal. The scale on the barrel is different for each size of syringe. The following table provides the usual volume measured by the smallest increments (marks) on the syringe. (The volumes provided could be wrong for your particular syringe -- please make sure before use.)

SIZE (IN CC) OF SYRINGE	VOLUME (IN CC) OF SMALLEST LINE ON THE SYRINGE
1 (tuberculin)	0.01 (1/100)
3	0.1 (1/10)
5	0.2 (2/10)
6	0.2 (2/10)
10	0.2 (2/10)
12	0.2 (2/10)
20	1.0
35	1.0
60	1.0

Notes on using a syringe

1. To make sure it works properly, move plunger up and down the barrel 2 or 3 times. If it does not move freely and tightly then it may not work -- you may need to test it with some sterile water before risking the medicine.
2. There are 2 types of syringe tips -- slip tip and locking-screw tip. The needle hub attaches here. Proper use of both tips require turning the needle hub onto the syringe tip in one direction and taking it off by turning the other way.
3. After determining the amount of medicine that will be removed from the bottle, pull the plunger back on the syringe to that mark on the barrel. The syringe is now filled with that amount of air. Push some or all of this air into the drug vial. This will help get the drug out by preventing a suction. One can inject a little air, remove some drug, inject some more air,

remove more drug ... until the volume of drug needed is inside the syringe. <u>CAUTION: do not inject more air into the vial than is necessary.</u>

4. Always aspirate after inserting the needle in an animal and look for blood in the tip of the syringe or in the hub of the needle. If blood is seen, then pull the needle out and push it in a new site. Aspirate again to make sure no blood is seen. A very bad allergic reaction will occur if a drug is injected into a blood vessel and it should have been administered IM or SQ.
5. If the drug leaks past the side of the rubber tip of the plunger, then the syringe is worn out and should not be used. If leakage is noticed during an injection, then push the plunger more slowly and gently. This may allow the injection to be finished without any more leakage.
6. Thick medications like the Penicillins are given more quickly and easily through the largest needle possible. This table provides some guidelines for needle selection.

	IM/SQ		IV/IP	
	SIZE RANGE (gauge)	LENGTHS (in inches)	SIZES	LENGTHS
CAT	25 – 21	5/8 – 1	25-22	5/8 – 1
DOG	25 – 20	"	25-18	"
GOAT SHEEP	22 – 18	1	22-16	3/4 – 1 1/2
PIG	21 – 18	1 – 1 1/2	22-18	1 – 1 1/2
BOVINE	20 – 16	1 – 1 1/2	20-12	1 – 1 1/2
HORSE	20 – 18	1 – 1 1/2	20-14	1 – 1 1/2
LLAMA	21 – 18	"	"	"
GUINEA PIG	25 – 22	5/8 – 1	NOT USED	
RABBIT	25 – 21	"	25-22	5/8 – 1
BIRDS	"	"	"	"

7. Frightened, nervous or vicious animals often jump or shake after the needle is placed causing the syringe and needle to fall out or the syringe hub to break. The following method may help when working with jumpy animals. Insert only the needle into the animal. After it has calmed down, attach the syringe and proceed with the injection.
8. Use sharp needles so that the pain associated with the needle insertion is minimized.

The following pages illustrate injection sites for cattle, sheep and goats, llamas, horses, poultry, rabbits and guinea pigs, cats, dogs, and pigs.

INJECTION SITES: OX

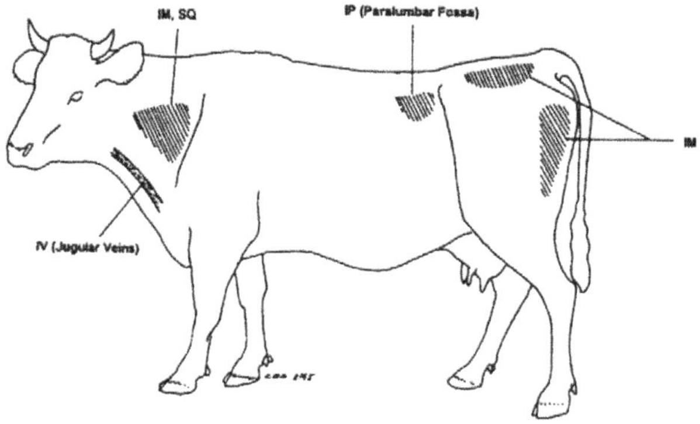

INTRAMUSCULAR INJECTION SITES: OX HINDQUARTERS

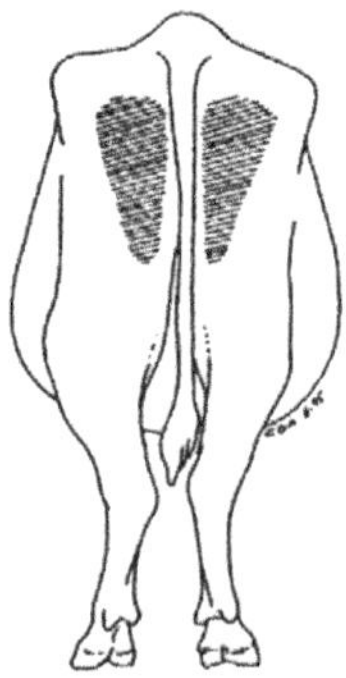

INTRAMUSCULAR INJECTION SITES: SHEEP OR GOATS

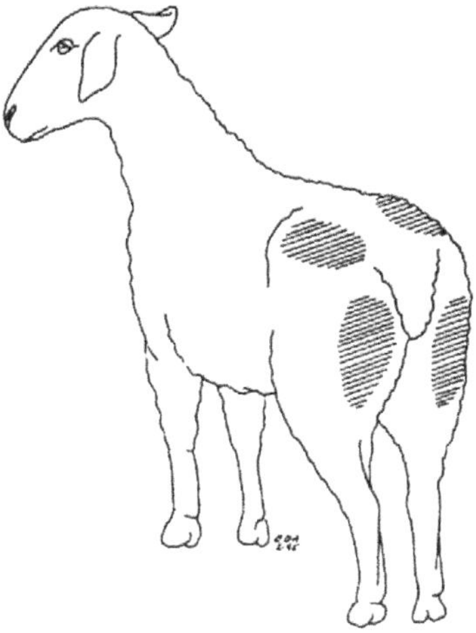

INJECTION SITES: SHEEP OR GOATS

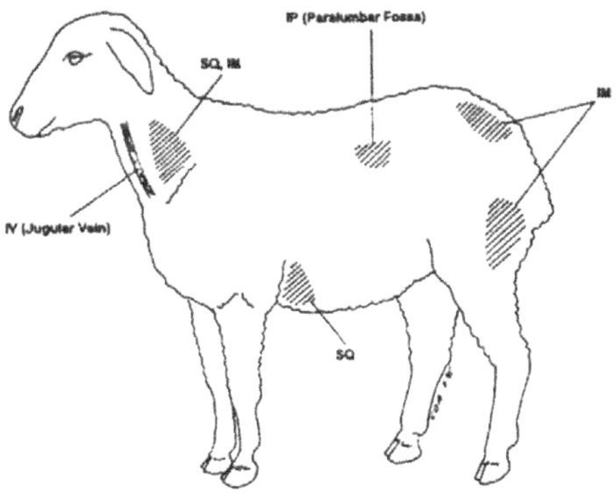

INJECTION SITES: LLAMA

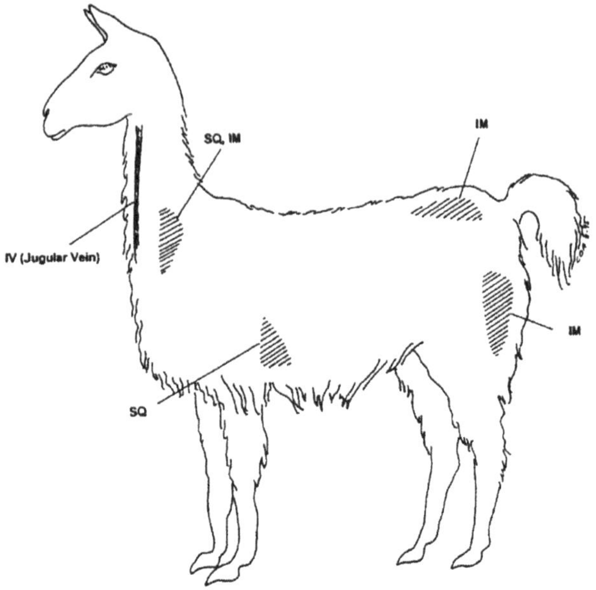

INJECTION SITES: HORSE

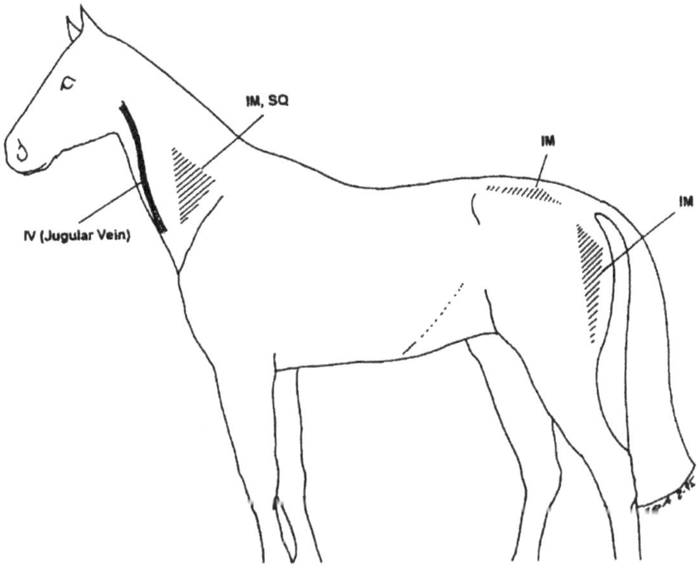

INJECTION SITES: HORSE

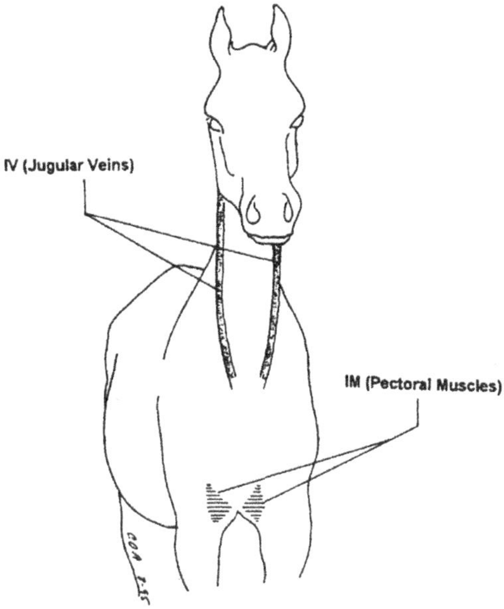

INTRAMUSCULAR INJECTION SITES: HORSE HINDQUARTERS

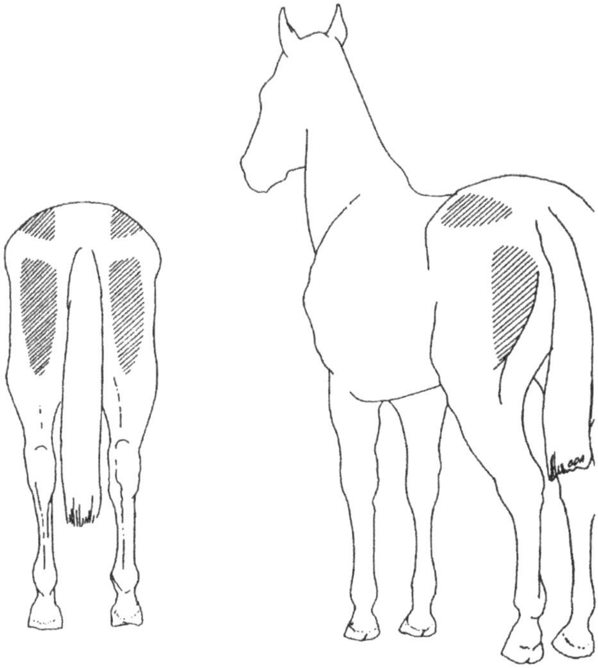

INJECTION SITES: POULTRY

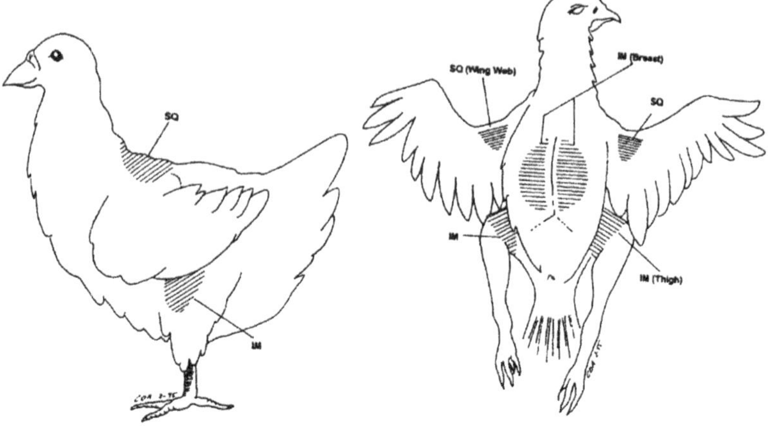

INJECTION SITES: RABBITS AND GUINEA PIGS

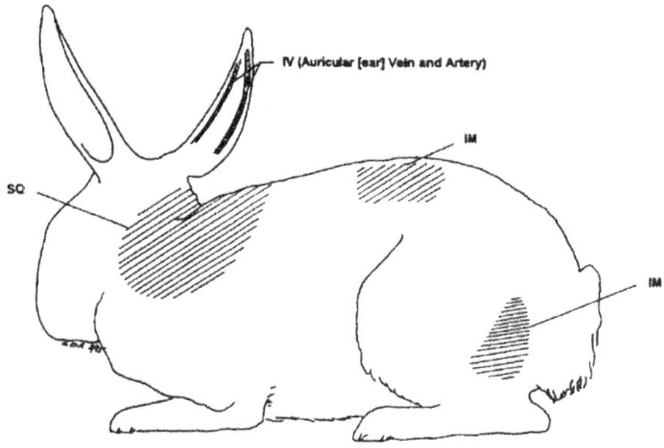

INJECTION SITES: DOGS AND CATS

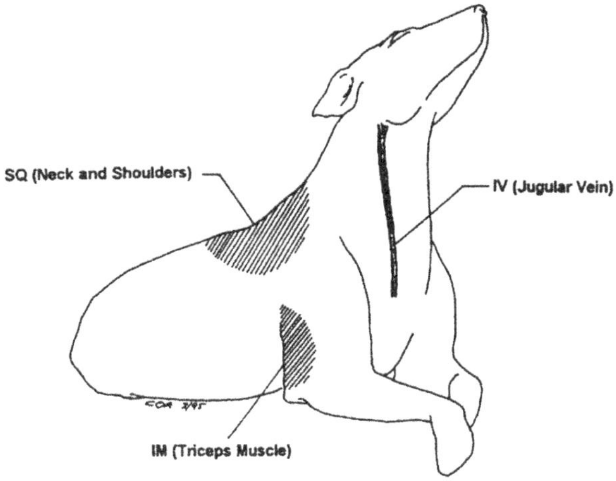

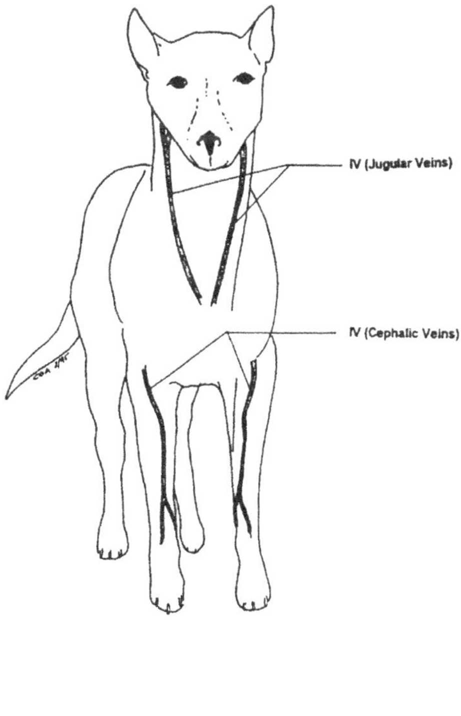

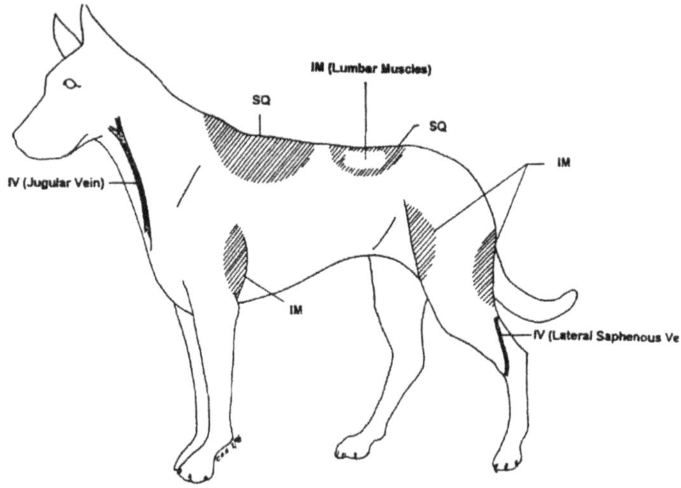

INJECTION SITES: PIG

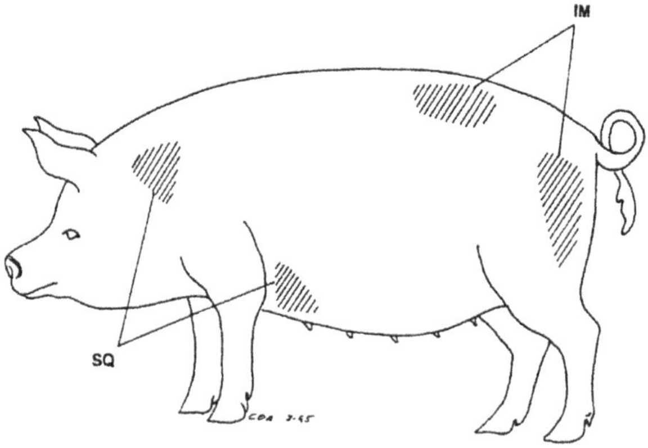

ORAL MEDICATIONS

Oral drugs may not be absorbed properly when given to an animal with gastrointestinal symptoms such as vomiting, diarrhea, constipation, or gastrointestinal stasis. Other symptoms such as ulcers or a swollen tongue may make swallowing difficult for an animal. Take care that the drug selected can be swallowed and that it is appropriate in those circumstances.

Adequate restraint is important for giving oral medicines. Tossing the head, backing away, or striking with a foot hinders their proper administration.

One method of dosing livestock by mouth is by pouring the medicine into the animals mouth from a long-necked bottle or a dose syringe. This method is called drenching. Drenching must be done carefully to keep the medicine from going into the lungs which can cause serious pneumonia and death.

To drench an animal, raise the head slightly to allow the medicine to run into the back of the throat. Don't raise it too high or the animal will have trouble swallowing. Place the medicine bottle (or dose syringe) into the side of the mouth so that the top rests on top of the tongue. Keep the bottle away from the teeth or the bottle may be broken. Pour the medicine slowly into the back of the mouth and allow the animal to swallow. If the animal starts to cough, stop giving the medicine, and let the head drop so that the medicine can be coughed out and not go into the lungs.

Another method of administering bitter or large volumes of liquids to animals is by passing a tube from the mouth or nose into the esophagus or stomach. THE TUBE MUST PASS TO THE STOMACH AND NOT TO THE LUNGS, for should the medicine be pushed into the lungs a severe pneumonia or death will occur. ALSO, DO NOT ALLOW THE ANIMAL TO CHEW ON THE TUBE. If the tube is chewed in two, then one piece may end up in the stomach and require surgery to be removed.

In order to be certain that the tube is indeed in the stomach do one or more of the following:

1) Watch the tube as it moves through the esophagus. The esophagus is a collapsing tube on the left side of the neck. Rarely will the esophagus be located on the right side of the neck. The trachea (windpipe) is always located in the center of the neck and is firm enough to be grasped or felt through the skin in the upper neck.
2) Suck on the <u>clean</u> end of the tube with your mouth. If air is able to be pulled continuously from the tube, then it is in the

trachea or lungs. If little to no air can be pulled out, then the tube is most likely in the esophagus or stomach.

3) Blow air into the tube while listening to the upper abdomen with an ear or stethoscope. If bubbling or gurgling is heard, then the tube is likely to be in the stomach.
4) If air comes out of the tube which smells sour, then it is likely to be in the stomach.
5) Usually a tube passing through the trachea or placed into the lungs will cause the animal to cough.
6) With experience the veterinary technician can feel a difference as the tube passes down the trachea as compared to the esophagus.

Some oral medications are bitter and will be spit out. Cats should not be given bitter liquids because they will salivate excessively. Forcing a liquid by holding the head up and pouring it down quickly may cause the animal to inhale the liquid leading to death or pneumonia. FORCING A LIQUID MUST BE DONE VERY CAREFULLY.

Tablets and capsules should be placed well back in the mouth, at the root of the tongue, to be swallowed. All animals will chew tablets not placed in or near the center of the root of the tongue. If a cat licks or chews a tablet then it may salivate excessively.

Pills and boluses should be given to livestock with a balling gun, a long handled instrument used to push the pills or boluses down the throat. To administer a pill or bolus using a balling gun, the animal is positioned as if drenching. The balling gun and bolus are placed over the tongue and back toward the throat, and the bolus is gently delivered into the back of the mouth. The head is held up slightly until the bolus is swallowed.

Drugs made to mix with food or water are used to treat large numbers of animals or birds. However, many sick animals or birds do not eat or drink enough to get the proper amount of drug to get well. Individual treatment assures each animal of bird receives the proper amount of medicine.

The following illustrate tools to deliver tablets, boluses or liquids.

Stomach Pump

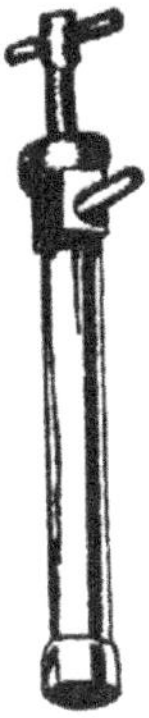
Pump handle
Attach stomach tube here
Siphon end goes into bucket containing fluids or medicine.

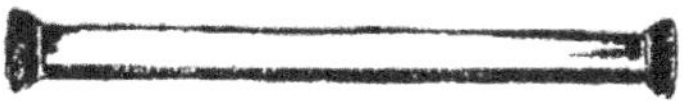

Frick cattle spectum

Plastic PVC pipe
for bolusing pills
(be sure ends are smooth)

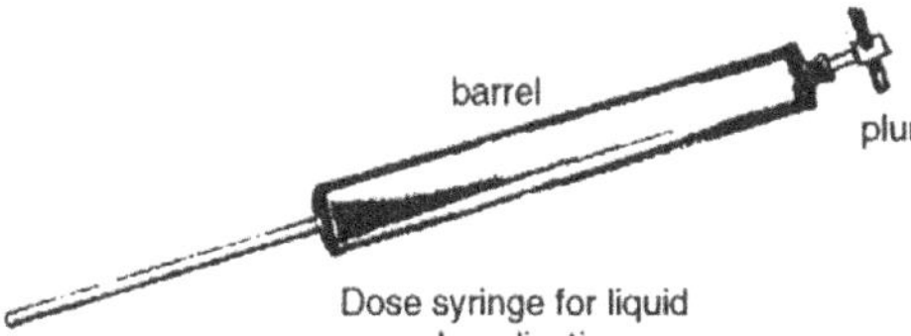

Dose syringe for liquid
oral medications

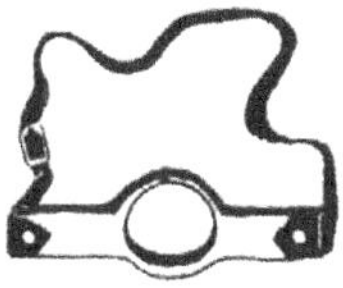

Stomach-tube speculum
prevents cattle from chewing tube as
it goes through the mouth.

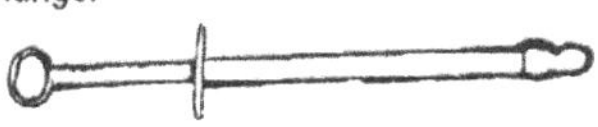
Hollow rubber tip holds pill
plunger

Small animal piller

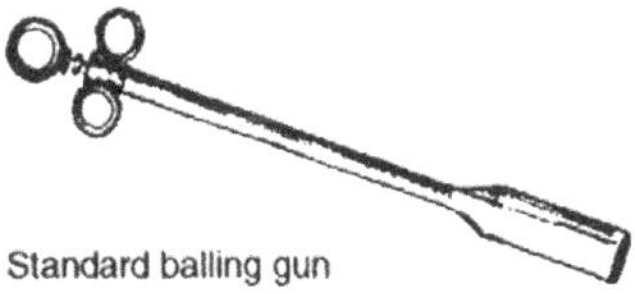

Standard balling gun

TOPICAL MEDICATIONS

The area to be treated should be clean of dirt and body fluids (pus, blood, etc.) prior to applying the medication. Topicals will not work when put on top of dirt or body fluids. Wounds which drain bloody fluids or pus must be washed frequently and new medication applied after each washing.

Animals can easily remove topicals by licking or rubbing. Bandaging, applying a collar, or tethering the head can prevent this.

Dirt, feces, leaves or grass will stick to topical ointments and liquids. A bandage may be needed.

Some topicals are toxic when swallowed. Some topicals can be absorbed in excess amounts through wounded skin leading to a toxicity. Applying too much topical medicine may do the same. These drugs can be harmful to the person applying them as well. FOLLOW THE LABEL INSTRUCTIONS REGARDING APPLICATION TECHNIQUE. TAKE THE NEEDED PRECAUTIONS.

Topical Insecticides

These are used to control flies, ticks, gnats, mosquitoes, mites and lice. They are supplied as sprays, dusts, dips, or pour-ons.

DUSTS can be applied by hand, through a shaker can or dust bag. A self-treatment dust bag can be made from 2 burlap sacks, one placed inside the other, containing 2 to 4 kilograms of insecticide dust. These should be protected from rain. They are easily refilled or replaced if needed. Animals should contact a self-treatment device at least every 2 to 3 days if not daily. They should be installed where animals routinely travel to insure regular contact. Dust bags should be hung in groups or 2 or more, spaced about 12.5 cm. apart and positioned so that the bottom of the bag hangs 45 to 60 cm. below the withers of adult animals.

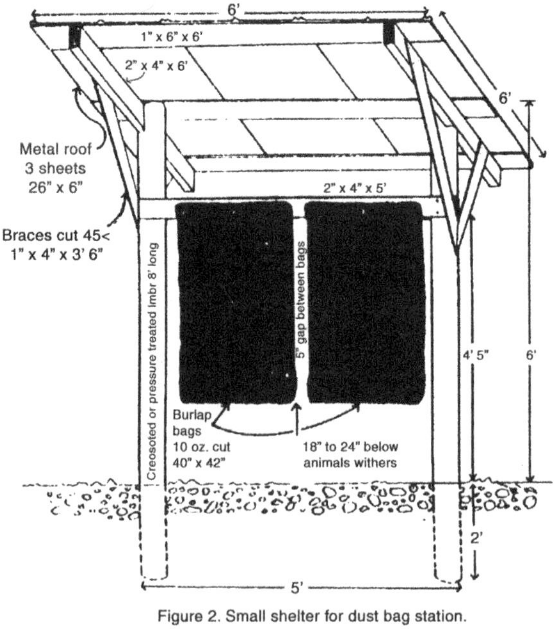

Figure 2. Small shelter for dust bag station.

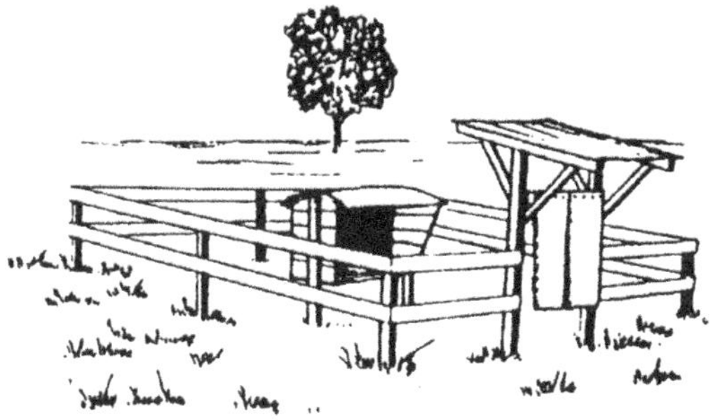

LIQUID INSECTICIDES for back rubber use come in ready-to-use formulas or as concentrates to be mixed with No. 2 diesel, kerosene or light mineral oil. DO NOT USE LUBRICATING OILS, SUCH AS AUTOMOBILE OIL, TO DILUTE INSECTICIDES FOR BACK RUBBER APPLICATION.

A simple oil-type back rubber can be made from a chain, cable, rope or 2 to 3 strands of wire twisted together, wrapped with several layers of securely tied burlap sacks and attached between trees. The middle of the back rubber should sag to 45 cm. from the ground. There should be enough looseness to the rubber that it easily gives way and rubs over the animal's back. Provide 6 m. of back rubber per 50-60 animals. The burlap is kept moist with the insecticide-oil solution. Animals should contact back rubbers with the same frequency as the dust bags, therefore they should be placed where animals routinely travel.

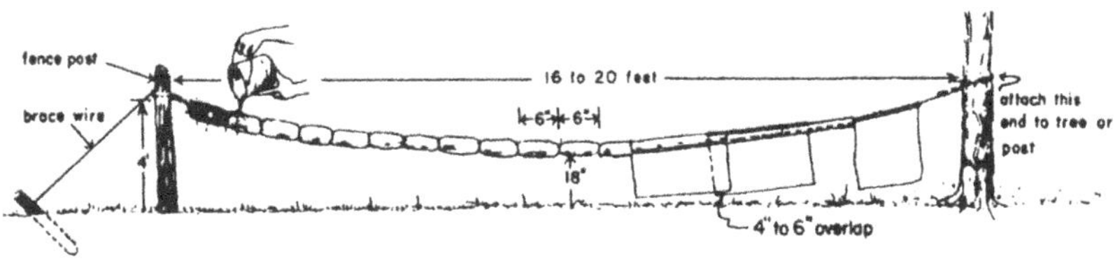

Figure 1. Simple type of homemade back rubber.

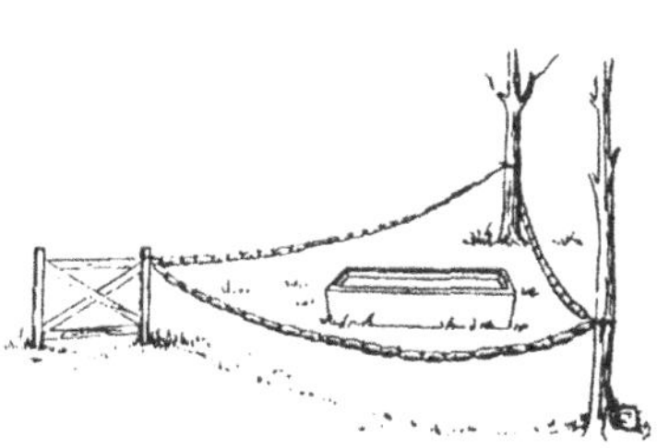

USEFULL INFORMATION TO KNOW

VOLUME: How much space or bulk something has. Used for measuring liquids.

1 teaspoon	= 5 cubic centimeters (cc) or 5 milliliters (ml)
3 teaspoons	= 1 tablespoon
1 tablespoon	= 15 cc/ml
2 tablespoons	= 30 cc/ml = one fluid ounce
8 ounces	= 1 cup = 240 cc/ml
2 cups	= 1 pint = 480 cc/ml
2 pints	= 1 quart = 32 fluid ounces
1 quart	= Approx. 1 liter (1000 cc/ml) (1 quart is just a little less than a liter)
4 quarts	= 1 gallon = Approx. 4000 cc/ml
1%	= 1 cm/100 ml

WEIGHTS: how heavy something is

16 ounces (oz)	= one pound (lb)
1 pound	= 454 grams (gm)
1000 grams	= 1 kilogram (kilo, kg)
1 kilogram	= 2.54 pounds
1 ounce	= 28 grams
1 gram	= 1000mg
1 grain (gr)	= 65 mg

METRIC MEASUREMENTS

1 milliiter (ml)	= 1 cubic centimeter (cc)
1000 ml	= 1 liter
1 gram (gm)	= 1000 milligrams (mg)
1 kilogram (kilo, kg)	= 2.2 pounds (lb)

To change centigrade to Fahrenheit multiply by 9/5 and add 32
To change Fahrenheit to centigrade subtract 32 and multiply by 5/9

SECTION 7

DRUG FORMULARY

DRUG FORMULARY

Randy C. Lynn, DVM, MS, DACVCP

The drug formulary is a listing of the drugs that are often used in animals. Important points about the type of drug, what it is used for, which animals can be given the drug, the dosage, route of administration, withdrawal times and precautions about drug interactions and possible adverse effects are included The formulary should only be consulted after the section of "Proper Drug Use" is read and understood. The drugs are grouped together by type and class. To find a specific drug quickly consult the index at the end of the book.

I am indebted to Rodney K. Frank, DVM, Ph.D., Pharmacia and Upjohn Inc., Kalamazoo, Michigan, and Thomas Powers, DVM, Ph.D., Professor Emeritus, the Ohio State University College of Veterinary Medicine for their guidance and editorial assistance. I owe special gratitude to Will Grimley, DVM and Leroy Dorminy, DVM without their help and encouragement, this chapter would not have been possible.

PROPER DRUG USE

Drug Selection:

Selection of the best drug to use should be made considering the type of animal, the condition that requires treatment, and which drugs are available and affordable. Veterinary clinical pharmacology is an immense area of study, this book contains only the most critical points that should be understood in order to use animal drugs safely and effectively. In developed countries, veterinarians spend many years learning the science of pharmacology and proper drug use before they are permitted to prescribe animal drugs. Users of this book may not have access to this type of training, and therefore should read the entire book, paying particular attention to the sections that deal with which drugs are most likely to be effective for treatment of animal conditions.

In most cases, a few drugs in each drug class will be adequate to meet the needs of local patients. To have a complete drug stock, you probably only need one anthelmintic, one injectable and one oral antibiotic in one or two antibiotic groups, one anti-inflammatory, one or two vitamin preparations and adrenaline to have a rather complete drug stock. A specific example of a well stocked drug case might include; ivermectin, Penicillin G injection, oxytetracycline injection, gentamicin injection, oral neomycin, an oral sulfonamide, dexamethasone, and injectable vitamin B complex. With these eight drugs most common animal conditions can be treated successfully. The practitioner should become thoroughly familiar with the selected drugs in their possession. Typically the source and availability of various drugs may change. One type of drug may be exchanged for another of the same type. For example, if one oral sulfa is not available, then a similar sulfa may be selected. If oral neomycin is unavailable, then substitute oral gentamicin (they are both aminoglycoside antibiotics).

In the remainder of this chapter animal drugs are grouped together by drug class, thus similar drugs are listed together. The list of drugs is long and contains drugs that are relatively inexpensive and others that are expensive. Expensive drugs are sometimes donated to practitioners in developing countries and information about those drugs is needed to allow them to be used to their fullest.

Withdrawal Period:

Drug withdrawal to prevent drug residues in meat and milk is very important subject for third world practitioners. Remember the old adage **"Above all, do no harm."** Many of the animals you treat will be used for human food, as meat or milk. When a drug is given to the live animal it goes throughout the body and is present in the flesh and milk of the animal until the body clears it from the system. If the animal is eaten or milk is consumed while the drug is still present the remaining drug can make people sick. In severe cases **the reaction can be fatal** to the person who eats the meat or milk. In developed countries there are very strict laws and systems in place to prevent drug residues in human food.

How to avoid drug residues; 1) Determine if the animal should be treated. If the animal is near normal slaughter age or weight and the drug is not critically needed to save the animals life or if the drug is needed to save the animal but is unlikely to keep the animal alive long enough for the entire withdrawal period then it may be better to slaughter the animal immediately rather than give the drug and make the animal unfit for human consumption. For example, if you have a calf that is just about ready to slaughter, but it has an infected foot that will require many days of antibiotic treatment and a prolonged withdrawal period. It may be better to slaughter the calf, and throw away the infected foot rather than to risk antibiotic therapy and throw away the whole animal.

2) If drug therapy is given, determine how long a time the drug must be withdrawn to prevent residues. The listed drug withdrawal

times are a general guide to the absolute **minimum time to wait after the last dose of drug is given**. If for example oxytetracycline is given to a calf at the dose of 10 mg/kg IM for 7 days, the calf should not be slaughtered until 18 days after the last dose which is 25 days (7 + 18 = 25) after the first dose was given. For milk to be used for human consumption the withdrawal period is 3 days. Be sure to consult the figures in this book and on the drug label; use whichever withdrawal period is longer! The withdrawal periods are determined at the label dose; if the drug is given at higher doses, or for longer durations of therapy then the withdrawal period should be increased as an extra margin of safety.

3) Identify the animal. Be sure to identify the animal to remind the owner that the animal in some way has been treated with drugs. Use a livestock crayon, paint marker, ear tag, purple wound spray or anything that will stay on for the duration of the treatment and withdrawal period. Owners can quickly forget that their animal was sick and has drug residues in the tissues.

4) Instruct the owner when it will be safe to consume or sell meat or milk from the animal. Tell the owner exactly what drugs you have given to their animal and how it will affect the meat and milk and for how long. Tell them exactly when the animal will be safe to eat or its milk safe to drink.

Following these four simple steps will help keep the human food supply free of any drug residues which can make people sick. Your job is to help supply people with safe animal food products that they need to survive and thrive.

Dewormers (Anthelmintics)

Anthelmintics are drugs that are used to remove worms and other internal parasites from animals. The drugs work by killing the parasite but not the host animal. Sometimes the wrong drug or wrong dose may poison the host animal. Be sure to choose the anthelmintic drug and calculate the dose carefully.

ABAMECTIN (Avomec)

Indications: Abamectin is a macrolide drug that has a broad spectrum of activity. It is effective against a wide range of internal and external parasites. The only disadvantage is cost.

Dosage and Route: Cattle - 0.2 mg/kg, SC[1]

Withdrawal Period: Cattle - Meat 30 days, Milk 30 days[1]

ALBENDAZOLE (Valbazen)

Indications: Albendazole is a broad spectrum benzimidazole anthelmintic for cattle and sheep which kills liver flukes, tapeworms, stomach worms, intestinal worms and lungworms. It is also used as a general dewormer in horses dogs and cats.

Dosage & Route:

Horses- 50 mg/kg by mouth for 2 days[2]
Cattle- 10 mg/kg by mouth[2]
Swine- 5-10 mg/kg by mouth[3]
Sheep- 7.5-15 mg/kg by mouth for adult liver flukes[3]
3 mg/kg by mouth for 35 days for prevention of liver flukes
Goats-7.5-15 mg/kg by mouth for adult liver flukes[3]
3 mg/kg by mouth for 35 days for prevention of liver flukes
Llama- 6.5 mg/kg by mouth[14]
Dogs- 25-50 mg/kg by mouth for 5 days[3]
Cats- 30 mg/kg by mouth for 6 days[3]

Withdrawal period:

Cattle - meat 27 days, do not use in milking cows[1]

Precautions: Do not give to female cattle in the first 45 days of pregnancy or within 45 days of breeding.

AMPROLIUM (Amprol, Corid)

Indications: Amprolium is a thiamine antagonist which inhibits the growth and reproduction of coccidia. It is used in calves to treat coccidiosis.

Dosage & Route:

Cattle- 5-10 mg/kg/day by mouth for 5 days[2]
Swine-25-65 mg/kg by mouth, 1-2 times daily for 3-4 days, or 100 mg/kg/day in food or water[3]
Sheep- 55 mg/kg by mouth daily for 19 days
Goats- 55 mg/kg by mouth daily for 19 days
Llama- 5 mg/kg by mouth for 3 weeks[14]
Dog- 100-200 mg/kg per day orally, 7-10 days

Withdrawal period: Cattle: 24 hours[2]

Precautions: High doses or prolonged administration can produce nerve damage. Administration of thiamine can counteract the effectiveness of amprolium. Do not use for more that 12 days in puppies.

BUNAMIDINE (Scolaban)

Indications: Bunamidine is an old drug that is used to kill tapeworms in dogs and cats.

Dosage and Route:

Dogs- 25-50 mg/kg by mouth[4]

Cats- 25-50 mg/kg by mouth[4]

Precautions: Vomiting and diarrhea may occur at the recommended dose. Sudden death may also occur on rare occasions.

CAMBENDAZOLE (Camvet)

Indications: Cambendazole is a broad spectrum dewormer.

Dosage and Route:

Horse- 20 mg/kg by mouth[4]

Cattle- 20 mg/kg by mouth[4]

Swine- 20-40 mg/kg by mouth[4]

Sheep- 20 mg/kg by mouth[4]

Withdrawal: Cattle- meat 21 days[4]

Precautions: Do not use in lactating dairy cows due to residues in the milk[4]

CLORSULON (Curatrem)

Indications: Kills liver flukes in cattle and sheep.

Dosage and Route:

Cattle-7 mg/kg by mouth, one dose[2]

Sheep-7 mg/kg by mouth, one dose[3]

Llamas- 7 mg/kg by mouth, one dose[3]

Camels- 7 mg/kg by mouth, every 60 days for 2 doses[14]

Withdrawal period: Cattle: 8 days for meat[2]

Precautions: Not to be used in lactating dairy cattle.

CLOSANTEL (Seponver, Razar)

Indications: Closantel kills flukes and worms when given by mouth or by injection.

Dosage and Route:

Cattle- 10 mg/kg by mouth; or 5 mg/kg SC[4]

Sheep- 10 mg/kg by mouth; or 5 mg/kg SC[4]

Withdrawal Period: Cattle- meat 28 days,

Sheep- meat 28 days[1]

DIAMPHENETHIDE

Indications: Diamphenethide kills liver flukes in sheep.
Dosage and Route: Sheep- 100 mg/kg by mouth[4]
Withdrawal Period: Sheep- meat 7 days[4]
Precautions: Do not give to sheep producing milk for human consumption.[4]

DICHLOROPHENE

Indications: Dichlorophene kills tapeworm in dogs and cats.
Dosage and Route: Dogs-200 mg/kg by mouth[4]
Cats- 200 mg/kg by mouth[4]
Precautions: May occasionally cause vomiting and diarrhea.

DICHLORVOS

Indications: Dichlorvos is available under many trade names including; Atgard, Cutter Dichlorvos Horse Wormer, and Task. Dichlorvos is an organophosphate chemical which has insecticidal properties when used externally and anthelmintic actions when used internally. In horses it is used to kill bots, strongyles and pinworms. In swine it is effective against roundworms and whipworms. In dogs the tablet form kills roundworms and hookworms, the capsule formulation is active against roundworms, hookworms and whipworms.

Dosage and Route:
Horse- Granules or paste 35 mg/kg by mouth
NOT RECOMMENDED IN FOALS[2]
Swine- 35 mg/kg by mouth[2]
Dog - 11-22 mg/kg by mouth[2]

Precautions: Since dichlorvos is an organophosphate chemical, toxicity can include; colic, salivation, diarrhea, slow heart rate, and breathing difficulties. Atropine and pralidoxime are antidotes. Keep away from food and children. Do not give to dogs with heartworms.

DIETHYLCARBAMAZINE

Indications: Diethylcarbamazine is most commonly used as a heartworm preventative for dogs. It may also be used in horses for treatment of filarial parasites like onchocercariasis.

Dosage and Route:
Horses- 1 mg/kg by mouth daily for 21 days for onchocerciasis[2]
Cattle- 22 mg/kg IM for 3 days; or
44 mg/kg IM once for *Dictyocaulus viviparous*[3]

Dogs- 6.6 mg/kg (3 mg/lb) by mouth every day during heartworm (mosquito) season; or 55-110 mg/kg by mouth for roundworms[3]

Precautions: Vomiting and diarrhea occasionally occur in dogs treated with diethylcarbamazine. Dogs harboring adult heartworm microfilaria will develop life-threatening reactions when given diethylcarbamazine. All dogs should be checked for microfilaria before beginning diethycarbamazine prophylaxis.

DISOPHENOL (DNP)

Indications: Disophenol (DNP) is an injectable dewormer for use in dogs, that is effective against hookworms.

Dosage and Route: Dog 10 mg/kg SC

Precautions: DNP injections frequently cause discomfort at the site of injection. The injectable solution produces a yellow stain if spilled on fabric or fur.[11]

EPSIPRANTEL (Cestex)

Indications: Epsiprantel is a tapewormer for use in dogs and cats.

Dosage and Route: Dog- 5.5 mg/kg by mouth[2]
Cat- 2.75 mg/kg by mouth[2]

Precautions: Do not use in puppies and kittens less than 7 weeks old.

FEBANTEL (Rintal)

Indications: Febantel is a broad-spectrum anthelmintic which is metabolized in the body into fenbendazole and oxfendazole. Febantel is most commonly used in horses against large and small strongyles, ascarids, and pinworms. It is effective against internal parasites of sheep. It is also used in dogs to remove roundworms, hookworms and whipworms.

Dosage and Route:

Horse- 6 mg/kg by mouth[2]
Cattle- 5-10 mg/kg by mouth[3]
Sheep- 5-10 mg/kg by mouth[3]
Dog- 10 mg/kg by mouth for 3 days[3]
Puppies-15 mg/kg by mouth for 3 days[3]
Cat- 10 mg/kg by mouth for 3 days[3]
Kittens-15 mg/kg by mouth for 3 days[3]

Withdrawal Period: Unknown

Precautions: When given to dogs and cats, febantel must be given for three days in a row to be effective.

FENBENDAZOLE (Panacur)

Indications: Fenbendazole is a broad-spectrum anthelmintic that is used in horses, swine, cattle, dogs and cats for a wide range of internal parasites. It is one of the most popular benzimidazole anthelmintics due to its safety and efficacy and due to the many formulations available including oral paste, oral granules, suspension and powder.

Dosage and Route:

Horse-5 mg/kg by mouth[2]; or 10 mg/kg by mouth for *Parascaris equorum*[2], or 50 mg/kg by mouth for *Stongyloides westeri*[2]

Cattle-5 mg/kg by mouth[2]; or 10 mg/kg by mouth for *Moniezia* and arrested *Ostertagia*[2]

Swine- 3 mg/kg by mouth for 3 consecutive days; or 5-10 mg/kg by mouth[3]

Sheep- 5 mg/kg by mouth for 3 days[3]

Camel- 4.5-15 mg/kg by mouth[14]

Llamas- 10-15 mg/kg by mouth[3]

Goats- 5 mg/kg by mouth for 3 days[3]

Dogs- 50 mg/kg by mouth daily for 3 days

Cats- 50 mg/kg by mouth daily for 5 days[3]

Rabbit-10 mg/kg by mouth every 14 days for 2 doses[14]

Withdrawal Period:

Cattle- meat 14 days[1], milk 4 days[1]

Sheep- meat 14 days[1]

Goats- meat 14 days[1], milk 1 day[1]

Precautions: Dogs, cats, and pigs must get the drug daily for three days in a row to be effective.

FLUBENDAZOLE

Indications: Flubendazole kills roundworms in pigs.

Dosage and Route: Swine-5 mg/kg by mouth; or 30 ppm in feed[4]

Withdrawal Period: Swine- meat 14 days[4]

IVERMECTIN (Ivomec, Zimectin)

Indications: Ivermectin is a macrolide drug that has the broadest spectrum of activity of any marketed antiparasite drug. Ivermectin is effective against a wide range of internal and external parasites. It is approved for use in more species of animal than any other antiparasite drug. The only disadvantage is cost.

Dosage and Route:

Horses-0.2 mg/kg by mouth[2]
Cattle-0.2 mg/kg by mouth or SC[2]
0.5 mg/kg pour-on (only use pour-on product for this route of application)[2]
Swine-0.3 mg/kg SC or IM
Sheep-0.2 mg/kg by mouth
Goat-0.2 mg/kg SC[14]
Llamas-0.2 mg/kg by mouth or injection[3]
African Buffalo- 0.2 mg/kg SC[14]
Camel-0.2 mg/kg SC[14]
Dogs-0.006 mg/kg by mouth monthly for heartworms[2].
0.05 mg/kg by mouth for removal of heartworm microfilariae[2]
0.2 mg/kg by mouth or by injection for intestinal worms[2]
Cats-0.2 mg/kg by injection for ear mites[2]
0.3 mg/kg by mouth or injection for intestinal worms[2]
Guinea Pig- 0.2-0.3 mg/kg SC[14]
Rabbit-0.2-0.4 by mouth, IM, SC[14]

Withdrawal Period:

Cattle-Meat 49 days, Do not use in milking cows[2]
Sheep-Meat 11 days.
Pigs-Meat 18 days.

Precautions: Do not give Collie dogs more than the 0.006 mg/kg dose as a fatal reaction may result. Do not give to dogs with heartworms.

LEVAMISOLE (Levasole, Ripercol, Totalon)

Indications: Levamisole is one of the standard anthelmintics that has been used effectively for many years. It is a broad spectrum drug that is commonly given by mouth, but special formulations are available for injection or pour-on

Dosage and Route:

Horses-8 mg/kg by mouth[2]
Cattle-8 mg/kg by mouth[2]
10 mg/kg using special pour-on product
6 mg/kg by SC[2]
Swine-8 mg/kg in water or feed
Sheep-8 mg/kg by mouth[3]
Goats-8 mg/kg by mouth[3]
Llamas-5-8 mg/kg by mouth[3]
Camels-5-8 mg/kg by mouth[3]
Dogs-10 mg/kg by mouth daily for 10 days for heartworm microfilaria; or
7-12 mg/kg by mouth daily for 3-7 days for lungworm[3]
Cats-20-40 mg/kg by mouth every other days for 6 treatments[3]

Withdrawal Period:

Cattle-meat 9 days, do not use in milking cows[2]
Sheep-meat 3 days
Swine-meat 9 days[3]

Precautions: Do not use at the same time as chloramphenicol. Toxic doses may produce signs similar to organophosphate toxicity; diarrhea, salivation, tremors, and foaming at the mouth. Atropine is somewhat helpful in treating an overdose.

LUXABENDAZOLE

Indications: Luxabendazole is a broad spectrum dewormer, that kills worms and flukes in sheep.

Dosage and Route:

Sheep-7.5 mg/kg by mouth; or[4]
10 mg/kg by mouth for flukes[4]

MEBENDAZOLE (Benzicare, Equiverm, Telmin)

Indications: Mebendazole powder, suspension, or paste is a broad spectrum anthelmintic most commonly used in horses, dogs, cats, sheep and swine.

Dosage and Route:

Horses-10-15 mg/kg by mouth; or
15-20 mg/kg by mouth for 5 days against lungworms[3]
Cattle-15 mg/kg by mouth[3]
Sheep-15 mg/kg by mouth[3]
Llamas- 22 mg/kg by mouth for 3 days[2]

Camels-22 mg/kg by mouth[14]
Dogs-22 mg/kg by mouth for 3 days[2]
Cats-22 mg/kg by mouth for 3 days[2]
Ferret-50 mg/kg by mouth twice a day for 2days[14]

Withdrawal: Sheep- meat 7 days[1]

Precautions: Mebendazole must be given daily for 3 days in a row to be effective in pigs, dogs and cats.

MILBEMYCIN D

Indications: Milbemycin D is approved in Japan to prevent heartworm infection in dogs.

Dosage and Route:

Dogs-1 mg/kg by mouth once every 30 days[4]

Precautions: Do not give to dogs that have heartworms it can produce a bad reaction.

MILBEMYCIN OXIME (Interceptor, Endovet)

Indications: Milbemycin oxime is a broad-spectrum dewormer and heartworm preventative for use in dogs and cats.

Dosage and Route:

Dogs- 0.5 mg/kg by mouth to remove worms, repeat once every 30 days to prevent Heartworms[2]
Cats-2 mg/kg by mouth to remove worms, repeat once every 30 days to prevent heartworms[2]

Precautions: Do not give to dogs that have heartworms it can produce a bad reaction.

MORANTEL TARTRATE (Nematel, Rumatel)

Indications: Morantel tartrate is a very safe anthelmintic for use in cattle, it may be fed to milking dairy cattle without any withholding period for the milk. It is available as a pellet or pre-mix for the feed, an oral bolus and a long-lasting bolus that releases drug for 90 days.

Dosage and Route:

Horses- 10 mg/kg by mouth[1]
Cattle- 10 mg/kg by mouth[3]
Sheep-10 mg/kg by mouth[3]

Withdrawal Period: Cattle-meat 30 days (Canada), 14 days (US)milk 0 days[3]

MOXIDECTIN (Cydectin)

Indications: Moxidectin is the latest new anthelmintic to enter the marketplace. It has very good broad-spectrum activity at very low doses.

Dosage and Route:

Horses- 0.2 mg/by IM; or 0.3 mg/kg by mouth; or
0.2 mg/kg pour-on (using the pour-on product)[1]
Cattle-0.2-0.4 mg/kg by mouth
0.2-0.3 mg/kg SC[1]
Sheep-0.2-0.4 mg/kg SC or
0.2 mg/kg by mouth[1]
Dogs-0.003 mg/kg by mouth for heartworm prevention[1]
0.15 mg/kg by intestinal parasites[1]

Withdrawal Period:

Cattle-meat 14 days, do not use in milk cows[1]
Sheep-meat 7 days[1]

Precautions: Do not give to dogs that are infected with heartworms.

NETOBIMIN (Hapadex)

Indications: Netobimin is metabolized in the body to the active metabolite albendazole.

Dosage and Route:

Cattle-7.5 mg/kg by mouth[4]
Sheep-7.5 mg/kg by mouth[4]

Withdrawal Period:

Cattle- meat 10 days, milk 3 days[4]
Sheep-meat 5 days[4]

Precautions: Do not treat cattle in the 7 weeks of pregnancy, or sheep in the first 3 weeks of pregnancy as it may kill or deform the fetus.[4]

NICLOSAMIDE

Indications: Niclosamide kills tapeworms in dogs, cats and sheep.

Dosage and Route:

Sheep-52 mg/kg by mouth[1]
Dogs- 150 mg/kg by mouth[4]
Cats-150 mg/kg by mouth[4]
Rabbit-100 mg/kg by mouth, 2 doses one week apart[14]

NITROSCANATE (Lopatol)

Indications: Nitroscanate kills roundworms, hookworms and tapeworms in dogs.

Dosage and Route: Dogs-50 mg/kg by mouth[4]

Precautions: Do not give to cats, it can produce temporary paralysis. It may cause vomiting in dogs.

NITROXYNIL (Trodax)

Indications: Nitroxynil kills flukes when injected into cattle and sheep.

Dosage and Route:

Cattle-10 mg/kg SC[4]

Sheep-10 mg/kg SC[4]

Withdrawal Period: Cattle- meat 30 days[4]

Sheep- meat 28 days[1]

Precautions: Do not use in dairy cattle producing milk for human consumption. Calculate the dose carefully because the toxic dose is only 4 times the recommended dose

OXANTEL

Indications: Oxantel kills whipworms in dogs. It is usually combined with pyrantel pamoate for broad spectrum activity.

Dosage and Route: Dogs-55 mg/kg by mouth[4]

OXFENDAZOLE (Benzelmin, Synanthic, Systamex)

Indications: Oxfendazole is a broad-spectrum benzimidazole that acts directly and also is changed into fenbendazole in the body. It is commonly used in both cattle and horses. It is only given by mouth or by a special syringe that injects the drug directly through the skin and into the rumen (Syntex Rumen Injector). Be sure to follow instructions closely when using the injectable route of administration.

Dosage and Route:

Horses-10 mg/kg by mouth[2]

Cattle-2.5-5 mg/kg by mouth or intra-ruminal injection[3]

Swine-3 mg/kg by mouth[3]

Sheep-5 mg/kg by mouth[3]

Goats-7.5 mg/kg by mouth[3]

Camels-4.5 mg/kg by mouth[114]

Withdrawal Period:

Cattle- meat 8 days, do not use in milking cattle[1]
Swine-meat 10 days[1]
Sheep-meat 10 days[1]
Goats-meat 10 days[1]

OXIBENDAZOLE (Anthelcide, Equipar)

Indications: Oxibendazole is a broad-spectrum benzimidazole that is apparently effective against some of the worms that have developed resistance to other benzimazoles.

Dosage and Route:

Horses-10 - 15 mg/kg by mouth[3]
Cattle- 10-20 mg/kg by mouth[3]
Swine- 15 mg/kg by mouth[3]
Sheep- 10-20 mg/kg by mouth[3]

Withdrawal period: Cattle- meat 9 days, milk 2 days[4]

OXYCLOZANIDE

Indications: Oxyclozanide kills adult liver flukes in cattle and sheep.

Dosage and Route:

Cattle-10-15 mg/kg by mouth[4]
Sheep-10-15 mg/kg by mouth[4]

Withdrawal Period: Cattle- meat 14 days, milk 0 days

Precautions: Calculate the dose carefully because the toxic dose is only 4 times the recommended dose.

PARBENDAZOLE

Indications: Parbendazole is a broad-spectrum dewormer which is also effective against lungworm.

Dosage and Route:

Horses-2.5 -20 mg/kg by mouth[4]
Cattle- 30 mg/kg by mouth[4]
Swine- 30 mg/kg by mouth[4]
Sheep- 20-30 mg/kg by mouth[4]

Withdrawal Period: Meat 6 days

Precautions: Do not give to pregnant animals, it can cause deformities at high doses.

PHENOTHIAZINE

Indications: Phenothiazine is a very old drug that still has utility against worms in large animals.

Dosage and Route:

Horses- 66 mg/kg by mouth, do not exceed 30 g total dose[5]

Cattle-220 mg/kg by mouth, do not exceed 60 g total dose[5]

Sheep-12.5 g by mouth for lambs under 20 kg
25 g by mouth for adult sheep[5]

Withdrawal Period: Meat 7 days[1]

Precautions: Phenothiazine is a photosensitizer which can cause sunburn in treated animals and in people exposed to the drug. Be certain to provide shade for the animals and the handler should wash up thoroughly after handling the drug.

PIPERAZINE (Citrate, Hexahydrate)

Indications: Piperazine is a dewormer that is very effective against roundworms in large and small animals that has been used for many years. It is not broad spectrum. It is not recommended in cattle, sheep and goats due to resistance of parasites in these species. Dose is calculated based upon the amount of piperazine base.

Dosage and Route:

Horses- 88-110 mg/kg of piperazine base by mouth[2]
Swine-110 mg/kg of piperazine base by mouth
Dogs-45-65 mg/kg of piperazine base by mouth[3]
Cats-45-65 mg/kg of piperazine base by mouth[3]
Gerbil-2-3 g/L drinking water for one week[14]
Guinea Pig- 2-5 g/L drinking water for one week[14]
Hamster-10 g/L drinking water [14]
Rabbit-200 mg/kg by mouth[14]
Chicken-250 mg/kg by mouth[14], or
1 g/L drinking water for three days[14]

Precautions: Toxic doses may cause tremors, seizures and weakness. Do not give to animals with liver or kidney disease.

PRAZIQUANTEL (Droncit)

Indications: Praziquantel is a very safe, narrow-spectrum anthelmintic which is very effective against tapeworms in dogs and cats.

Dosage and Route:

Sheep- 10-15 mg/kg by mouth[3]
Goats- 10-15 mg/kg by mouth[3]
Llamas- 5 mg/kg by mouth[3]
Camels-10 mg/kg by mouth[14]
Dogs- 2.5-7.5 mg/kg by mouth or injected[2]
Cats- 2.5-7.5 mg/kg by mouth or injected[2]

PYRANTEL PAMOATE (Nemex, Strongid)

Indications: Pyrantel pamoate is a moderately broad-spectrum anthelmintic that is very safe to use. It is one of the most widely used dewormers for dogs and cats. Pyrantel does not work against whipworms.

Dosage and Route:

Horses- 20 mg/kg by mouth[4]
Swine- 6.6 mg/kg by mouth[14]
Camels-18 mg/kg by mouth[14]
Dogs- 5-15 mg/kg by mouth[2]
Cats- 10-20 mg/kg by mouth[2]
Llamas- 18 mg/kg by mouth[2]

Precautions: Do not use at the same time as piperazine, as toxicity may result.

PYRANTEL TARTRATE (Banminth)

Indications: A moderately broad spectrum anthelmintic that is very effective and very safe. It is the large animal cousin to pyrantel pamoate.

Dosage and Route:

Horse-14.4 mg/kg by mouth daily for control of worms[2]
Cattle- 25 mg/kg by mouth[2]
Swine- 22 mg/kg by mouth[3]
Sheep- 25 mg/kg by mouth
Goats- 25 mg/kg by mouth

Withdrawal Period: Swine- meat 1 day[3]

RAFOXANIDE

Indications: Rafoxanide kills flukes when given by mouth or by subcutaneous injection.

Dosage and Route: Cattle-7.5 mg/kg by mouth,
3 mg/kg SC[4]
Sheep- 7.5 mg/kg by mouth[4]

Withdrawal Period: Cattle-meat 28 days[4]

Precautions: Do not use in cattle producing milk for human consumption.

THENIUM CLOSYLATE (Canopar)

Indications: Thenium closylate kills hookworms in dogs.

Dosage and Route: Dogs-250 mg by mouth twice daily for dogs that weigh (5-10 pounds) 2.27-4.54 kg[2] 500 mg by mouth once for dogs that weigh more than (10 pounds) 4.54 kg[2]

Precautions: Use with caution in Airedales and Collie dogs. Vomiting occurs in about 20% of the dogs treated. Re-dose if vomiting occurs within 2 hours.

THIABENDAZOLE (TBZ, Equizole, Omnizole)

Indications: Thiabendazole was the first modern broad-spectrum dewormer. It is very effective and has been used effectively for many years. It is available in a wide range of formulations including; suspension, bolus, paste, feed block, feed premix and pellets.

Dosage and Route:
Horses- 50-100 mg/kg by mouth[3]
Cattle- 50-100 mg/kg by mouth[3]
Swine- 50-75 mg/kg by mouth[3]
Sheep- 50-100 mg/kg by mouth[3]
Goats- 66 mg/kg by mouth[3]
Llamas- 50-100 mg/kg by mouth daily for 1-3 days[3]
Camels-66 mg/kg by mouth[14]
Dogs- 50 mg/kg by mouth daily for three days
Rabbits-100-200 mg/kg by mouth[14]

Withdrawal Period: Cattle-meat 3 days, milk 4 days[3]
Sheep-meat 30 days[3]
Goats-meat 30 days[3]

THIOPHANATE

Indications: Thiophanate is metabolized in the body to the active metabolite lobendazole, it provides broad spectrum activity against worms in livestock.

Dosage and Route:

Cattle- 50 mg/kg by mouth[4]
Swine- 5-12 mg/kg by mouth for 14 days[4]
Sheep- 50 mg/kg by mouth[4]

Withdrawal Period: Cattle- meat 7 days[4]

TRICLABENDAZOLE (Fasinex)

Indications: Triclabendazole is very effective in killing liver flukes in cattle, sheep and goats. It is particularly effective against young flukes.

Dosage and Route:

Cattle- 12 mg/kg by mouth[4]
Sheep- 10 mg/kg by mouth[4]
Goats- 10 mg/kg by mouth[4]

Withdrawal Period: Cattle-Meat 28 days[4]

Precautions: Do not give to animals producing milk for human consumption. It is toxic to fish, keep out of streams, rivers and lakes.

TRICHLORFON

Indications: Trichlorfon is an organophosphate that can be used as a pour-on to control external parasites or can be given by mouth for control of internal parasites. It is especially useful for removing bots in horses. Because it is an organophosphate the dose should be calculated carefully. Oral solutions must be given to horses by stomach tube.

Dosage and Route:

Horses- 10 mg/kg by mouth for bots
40 mg/kg by mouth for other worms[2]
Cattle-15 ml of an 8% pour-on solution per 100 kg of body weight for grubs[3]
44-110 mg/kg by mouth for worms
Swine- 50 mg/kg by mouth[4]
Sheep- 44-110 mg/kg by mouth for worms

Withdrawal Period: Cattle- meat 21 days after pour-on[3]

Precautions: Do not use at the same time as other organophosphate insecticides or dewormers. Toxicity may include diarrhea, colic, or incoordination. Antidotes are atropine and pralidoxime (2PAM).

Antibiotics

Proper Antibiotic Use: Antibiotics are the most often overused and abused therapeutic agents used in animals. This overuse and abuse concerns many experts because of the potential danger of creating bacteria that are resistant to antibiotics and creating harmful residues in our food. Bacteria which are resistant to antibiotics make treatment of animals and people more difficult when they are faced with a severe life-threatening infection. Residues of antibiotics and other drugs in meat, milk and eggs can produce sickness in people that eat these foods. For these reasons it is important to limit the use of antibiotics to those animals that need them and to make sure that all who use antibiotics for treatment of food producing animals observe the proper withdrawal periods.

Choosing the best antibiotic: Many kinds of antibiotics are available and they differ widely in the types of bacteria that they work against and in their ability to penetrate into different tissues. Some antibiotics work well when combined with another antibiotic and some antibiotics will interfere with others so that there is no benefit to the sick animal. The simplest way to understand antibiotic use is to group similar antibiotics together into several broad groups. The main groups of antibiotics are the penicillins and cephalosporins, aminoglycosides, tetracyclines, and sulfas. Several other smaller groups are not included in this formulary but are covered in veterinary textbooks.

Penicillin and Cephalosporin Group

This group includes penicillin, amoxicillin, ampicillin, cephalexin, ceftiofur and others. They kill bacteria (bactericidal) by breaking the outer wall of the bacteria. They are very effective against common gram positive bacteria. Penicillins and cephalosporins are the safest of the antibiotics. On rare occasions they may cause an allergic reaction which can be fatal if not treated quickly with epinephrine. They give good drug levels in the respiratory and urinary tract. Penicillins and cephalosporins are often the first antibiotics used if the type of bacteria is unknown. They work especially well when combined with aminoglycoside antibiotic drugs. They should not be combined with tetracyclines, sulfas or chloramphenicol. Penicillins are rather inexpensive but cephalosporins can be quite expensive.

Important note: Most **injectable penicillins must be stored in a refrigerator** or on ice. This may prevent their use in some settings. Most are probably good to use for a few days at room temperature then should be discarded.

Aminoglycoside Group

This group includes streptomycin, gentamicin, kanamycin, neomycin and others. Aminoglycosides kill bacteria by disturbing the chemical machinery inside the bacteria. They are very effective against common gram negative bacteria. Aminoglycosides must be used with caution because of toxic side effects to the hearing and kidneys. They do not move across biological barriers. If given by mouth it stays in the gut; if injected it stays in the internal tissues. Some aminoglycisides like neomycin are very effective in treating diarrhea (scours) in baby animals. The injectable aminoglycosides are often reserved for more serious infections and are commonly used in combination with penicillins and cephalosporins. Injectable aminoglycosides have very long withdrawal periods Aminoglycosides should not be combined with tetracycline, sulfas or chloramphenicol.

Tetracycline Group

This group includes tetracycline, oxytetracycline, chlortetracycline and others. Tetracyclines inhibit the growth of bacteria so that the treated animal has a chance to overcome the infection. They also disturb the chemical machinery inside the bacteria. They move very well into the liver, respiratory tract and skin. Tetracyclines can be given by mouth, injection or externally (topically) to the eye. They should not be given to horses, because they can produce a fatal gastrointestinal condition (pseudomembranous colitis). If given to young growing animals and children, they produce a permanent discoloration and staining of the teeth. They can also produce liver and kidney damage. They are inexpensive and readily available. Do not combine with any other antibiotics.

Sulfa Group

This group includes many antibiotics that start with the name "sulfa" like sulfamethazine and sulfadimethoxine. This class of antibiotics has been around since the 1930s. They inhibit bacterial growth, are well absorbed and move well into most tissues of the body. Sulfas can be given by mouth, injection or externally when treating wounds. They are most effective when given with "potentiators" like trimethoprim or ormetoprim which make them much more effective. Sulfas should not be combined with any other antibiotics.

Deciding which antibiotics to use

Under conditions where there is no access to facilities for conducting bacterial culture and sensitivity empirical therapy is the only practical way to proceed. Empirical therapy means that an antibiotic should be selected based on the probability that it will most likely treat the condition at hand. The following list is an attempt to make selection easier. If the first choice does not seem to work after 3-5 days, then move to another in the list. When switching to another antibiotic, it is probably better to choose an antibiotic from another group. For example to the penicillin is not working it is probably better to try a an antibiotic from another group.

(Note: Pen = penicillin and cephulosprin group, Tet = tetracycline group, Amin = aminoglycoside group, Sulf = sulfa group, Chlor = chloramphenicol)

Horse and Donkey

Condition	First Choice	Second Choice
Pneumonia	Pen, Amin	Sulfa[6]
Diarrhea	Pen, Amin (oral)	Sulfa[6]
Genitourinary	Pen	Amino[6]
Other Soft Tissues	Pen	Sulfa[6]

Cattle

Condition	First Choice	Second Choice
Pneumonia	Pen, Tet	Sulfa, Amin[6]
Diarrhea	Amin (oral)	Sulfa[6]
Genitourinary	Pen	Amin, Sulfa[6]
Mastitis	Pen	Tet, Sulfa[6]
Other Soft Tissue	Pen	Tet[6]

Swine

Condition	First Choice	Second Choice
Pneumonia	Pen	Tet[6]
Diarrhea	Amin (oral)	Sulfa, Tylosin[6]
Genitourinary	Pen	Tet[6]
Skin	Pen	Amin[6]

Sheep and Goats

Condition	First Choice	Second Choice
Pneumonia	Tet	Sulfa, Tylosin[6]
Diarrhea	Amin	Sulfa[6]
Genitourinary	Tet	Pen, Amin, Sulfa[6]
Mastitis	Pen	Amin, Tet, Sulfa[6]
Other Soft Tissue	Pen	Tet[6]

Dogs and Cats

Condition	First Choice	Second Choice
Pneumonia	Pen, Sulfa	Amin, Tet[6]
Diarrhea	Pen, Amin (oral)	Sulfa, Chloro[6]
Genitourinary	Pen	Sulfa[6]
Other Soft Tissue	Pen	Sulfa[6]
Skin	Chloro	Erythro, Sulfa

ANTIBIOTIC DRUGS (Listed by Group)

Penicillin and Cephalosporin Group

AMOXICILLIN (Amoxi-Tab, Amoxi-Drop, Amoxi-Jet, Amoxil)

Indications: See "penicillin and cephalosporin group" above.

Dosage and Route:

Horses- 10-22 mg/kg IM, IV, 3-4 times daily
20 mg/kg by mouth 4 times daily[2]

Cattle- 11 mg/kg IM, SC once a day[2]; or
10-20 mg/kg by mouth, twice daily in young (non-ruminating) calves[2]; or 62.5 mg per quarter by intramammary infusion[2].

Dogs- 10-20 mg/kg by mouth or SC, 2 times daily[2]

Cats- 10-20 mg/kg by mouth or SC, twice daily[2]

Ferret- 10-20 mg/kg by mouth or SC, twice daily[14]

Chicken-55-110 mg/kg by mouth 2-3 times daily[14]

Withdrawal Period:

Cattle-Injected- meat 25 days, milk 4 days[2] Oral in calves- meat 20 days[2],
Intramammary fusion- milk 2.5 days[2], meat 12 days[2].

Precaution: Do not give to small herbivores, like rabbits and guinea pigs.

AMOXICILLIN/ Clavulonic acid (Clavamox, Clavulox)

Indications: See "penicillin and cephalosporin group" above. Amoxicillin in combination with a potentiator that prevents the bacteria from inactivating the antibiotic.

Dosage and Route:

Dogs- 10-20 mg/kg (amoxicillin) by mouth, 2 times daily[3]
Cats- 10-20 mg/kg (amoxicillin) by mouth, 2 times daily[3]

AMPICILLIN (Polyflex, Albipen)

Indications: See "penicillin and cephalosporin group" above.

Dosage and Route:

Horses- 11-22 mg/kg IM, IV, 2-3 times daily[2]
Cattle- 5-12 mg/kg IM once daily[2]
Swine-5-12 mg/kg IM once daily[2]
Llama-11 mg/kg IV, 3 times daily[14]
Dogs- 22 mg/kg, by mouth, 3 times daily[2]; or 11- 22 mg/kg, SC, IM, 3-4 times daily[2]
Cats-22 mg/kg, by mouth, 3 times daily[2]; or 11-22 mg/kg, SC, IM, 3-4 times daily[2]
Ferret-10 mg/kg IM, 2 times daily, or 20 mg/kg SC, 2 times daily, or 20 mg/kg by mouth, 2 times daily[14]

Withdrawal Period: Cattle- meat 6 days, milk 2 days[2]

CARBENICILLIN

Indications: See "penicillin and cephalosporin group" above.

Dosage and Route:

Horses- foals 100 mg/kg IV, 3-4 times daily[3]
Dogs- 15 mg/kg, by mouth or IV 3 times daily[3]
Cats- 15 mg/kg, by mouth or IV 3 times daily[3]

CEFACLOR (Ceclor)

Indications: See "penicillin and cephalosporin group" above.

Dosage and Route:

Horses- 20-40 mg/kg by mouth, 3 times daily[2]
Dogs- 4-20 mg/kg by mouth, 3 times daily[2]
Cats- 4-20 mg/kg by mouth, 3 times daily[2]

CEFADROXIL (Cefa-Tabs, Cefa-Drops)

Indications: See "penicillin and cephalosporin group" above.

Dosage and Route:

Horses- 22 mg/kg by mouth, twice daily[2]
Dogs-22 mg/kg by mouth, twice daily[2]
Cats- 22 mg/kg by mouth, twice daily[2]

CEFAMANDOLE

Indications: See "penicillin and cephalosporin group" above.

Dosage and Route:

Horses-10-30 mg/kg IM, IV, every 4-8 hours[2]
Dogs- 6-40 mg/kg IM, 3-4 times daily[2]
Cats- 6-40 mg/kg IM, 3-4 times daily[2]

CEFAZOLIN (Ancef, Kefzol)

Indications: See "penicillin and cephalosporin group" above.

Dosage and Route:

Horses-15 mg/kg IM, IV, 2-3 times daily[2]
Cattle- 22 mg/kg IM, 3 times daily[2]
Dogs- 5-15 mg/kg IM, 3-4 times daily[2]
Cats- 5-15 mg/kg IM, 3-4 times daily[2]
Chicken-11-55 mg/kg IM, 2-3 times daily[14]

Withdrawal period: Cattle- meat 30 days[2]

CEFONICID

Indications: See "penicillin and cephalosporin group" above.

Dosage and Route:

Horses- 10-15 mg/kg IM, IV once daily[2]

CEFOPERAZONE

Indications: See "penicillin and cephalosporin group" above.

Dosage and Route:

Horses- 30-50 mg/kg IM, IV, 2-3 times daily[2]

CEFORANIDE

Indications: See "penicillin and cephalosporin group" above.

Dosage and Route:

Horses- 5-10 mg/kg IM, IV 2 times daily[2]

CEFOTAXIME (Claforan)

Indications: See "penicillin and cephalosporin group" above.

Dosage and Route:

Horses- 25-50 mg/kg IM, IV, 2-3 times daily[2]
Dogs- 20-80 mg/kg IM, IV, SC, 3 times daily[2]
Cats- 20-80 mg/kg IM, IV, 3 times daily[2]

CEFOXITIN

Indications: See "penicillin and cephalosporin group" above.

Dosage and Route:

Horses- 30-40 mg/kg IM, 3-4 times daily[2]
Dogs- 6-20 mg/kg IM, SC 3 times daily[2]
Cats- 6-20 mg/kg IM, 3 times daily[2]

CEFTAZIDIME

Indications: See "penicillin and cephalosporin group" above.

Dosage and Route:

Horses- 25-50 mg/kg IM, IV, twice daily[2]
Dogs- 25 mg/kg IM, SC 2-3 times daily[2]
Cats- 25 mg/kg IM, SC 2-3 times daily[2]

CEFTIOFUR

Indications: See "penicillin and cephalosporin group" above.

Dosage and Route:

Horses-1-2 mg/kg IM, 1-2 times daily[2]
Cattle-1 mg/kg IM, once daily[2]
Swine-1.1-2.2 mg/kg IM[14]
Llama-1 mg/kg SC, 2 times daily, or
2-5 mg/kg IM, IV, 2 times daily[14]
Camel-2.2 mg/kg IV, once daily[14]
Chicken-0.08-0.2 mg total dose, SC[14]

Withdrawal period: Cattle- meat 0 days, milk 0 days (Canada)[2]

CEFTIZOXIME

Indications: See "penicillin and cephalosporin group" above.

Dosage and Route:

Horses- 25-50 mg/kg IM, IV, 2-3 times daily[2]

CEFTRIAXONE

Indications: See "penicillin and cephalosporin group" above

Dosage and Route:

Horses- 25-50 mg/kg IM, IV, twice daily[2]

CEFUROXIME AXETIL

Indications: See "penicillin and cephalosporin group" above.

Dosage and Route:

Horses- 25-50 mg/kg IM, IV, 3 times daily[2]
250-500 mg/kg by mouth, twice daily[2]

CEPHALEXIN (Keflex)

Indications: See "penicillin and cephalosporin group" above.

Dosage and Route:

Horses- 10-30 mg/kg by mouth, 3-4 times daily[2]
Goats-30 mg/kg, SC[14]
Dogs-10-30 mg/kg by mouth, 2-4 times daily[2]
Cats- 10-30 mg/kg by mouth, 2-4 times daily[2]
Rabbit-15 mg/kg, SC, 2 times daily[14]
Guinea Pig- 15 mg/kg, IM, 2 times daily[14]
Chicken-55-110 mg/kg by mouth, 2 times daily[14]

CEPHALORIDINE

Indications: See "penicillin and cephalosporin group" above.

Dosage and Route:

Horses- 10 mg/kg IM, SC, twice daily[2]
Cattle-10 mg/kg IM, SC, twice daily[2]
Swine-10 mg/kg IM, SC, twice daily[2]
Gerbil-30 mg/kg IM, twice daily[14]
Guinea Pig- 10-25 mg/kg IM, SC twice daily[14]
Hamster-30 mg/kg IM, twice daily[14]
Rabbit-10-25 mg/kg IM, SC, 2-3 times daily[14]

CEPHALOTHIN

Indications: See "penicillin and cephalosporin group" above.

Dosage and Route:

Horses- 20-40 mg/kg IM, IV, 3-4 times daily[2]
Cattle- 55 mg/kg SC, 4 times daily[3]
Dogs- 20-35 mg/kg IM, IV, SC, 3-4 times daily[2]
Cats- 20-35 mg/kg IM, IV, SC, 3-4 times daily[2]
Rabbit-12.5 mg/kg IM, 4 times daily[14]

CEPHAPIRIN (Cefa-Dri, Cefa-Lak)

Indications: See "penicillin and cephalosporin group" above.

Dosage and Route:

Horses-30 mg/kg IV, IM, every 4-6 hours[2]

Cattle-300 mg of cephapirin benzathine or 200mg of cephapirin sodium by intramammary infusion into each quarter[2]

Dogs- 20-30 mg/kg IM, IV, SC, 3 times daily[2]

Cats- 20-30 mg/kg IM, IV, SC, 3 times daily[2]

Withdrawal Period: Cattle-Cephapirin benzathine; meat 42 days, milk discarded for 3.5 days after calving[2]

Cephapirin sodium; meat 4 days[2], milk discarded for 4 days[2]

Precautions: The benzathine infusion should only be used in dry cows.

CLOXACILLIN (Orbenin, Dariclox, Dri-clox)

Indications: See "penicillin and cephalosporin group" above.

Dosage and Route:

Cattle-500 mg of cephapirin benzathine; or 200 mg of cephapirin sodium by intramammary infusion into each quarter[2]

Dogs- 10-40 mg/kg by mouth or IM 3-4 times daily[3]

Cats- 10-40 mg/kg by mouth or IM 3-4 times daily[3]

Withdrawal Period:

Cattle-Cephapirin benzathine; meat & milk 30 days[2], Cephapirin sodium; meat 10 days, milk discarded for 2 days (2.5 days Canada)[2].

Precautions: The benzathine infusion should only be used in dry cows.

DICLOXACILLIN

Indications: See "penicillin and cephalosporin group" above.

Dosage and Route:

Dogs-11-25 mg/kg by mouth 3 times daily[3]

Cats-11-25 mg/kg by mouth 3 times daily[3]

HETACILLIN (Hetacin-K)

Indications: See "penicillin and cephalosporin group" above. Hetacillin is metabolized in the body to ampicillin, the active metabolite.

Dosage and Route:

Cattle-5-15 mg/kg SC, IM, twice daily; or
62.5 mg per quarter, by intramammary infusion
Swine-5-15 mg/kg SC, IM, twice daily[2]
Dogs- 10-40 mg/kg by mouth, twice daily[2]
Cats- 50 mg by mouth, twice daily[2]

Withdrawal Period: Cattle- intramammary infusion, milk 3 days, meat 10 days[2]

NAFCILLIN

Indications: See "penicillin and cephalosporin group" above. Nafcillin is similar to cloxacillin and oxacillin. It is very effective against bacteria that are resistant to penicillin.

Dosage and Route:

Horses- 10 mg/kg IM, 3 times daily[2]
Dogs- 10 mg/kg by mouth, IM 4 times daily[2]
Cats- 10 mg/kg by mouth, IM 4 times daily[2]

Precautions: Naficillin can produce vomiting, diarrhea and rashes.

OXACILLIN

Indications: See "penicillin and cephalosporin group" above.

Dosage and Route:

Horses- Foals 20-30 mg/kg IV, 4 times daily [3]
Adults 25-50 mg/kg IM,IV, 2 times daily[3]
Dogs- 20-40 mg/kg by mouth, 3 times daily[3]
Cats- 20-40 mg/kg by mouth, 3 times daily[3]

Withdrawal Period: Cattle-intramammary infusion, milk 3 days, meat 10 days[3]

PENICILLIN G (sodium or potassium)

Indications: See "penicillin and cephalosporin group" above.

Dosage and Route:

Horses-10,000-50,000 IU/kg IM, IV, 4 times daily[2]
Cattle-10,000-50,000 IU/kg IM, IV, 4 times daily[2]
Dogs- 20,000 IU/kg, IM, SC, every four hours[2]
Cats- 20,000 IU/kg, IM, SC, every four hours[2]

Withdrawal Period: Note: effective doses greatly exceed the labeled dose, therefore the label withdrawal period must be longer than the label requires. Cattle-IM dosing, meat 21 days[2] SC dosing, meat 42 days[2]

PENICILLIN G (benzathine)

Indications: See "penicillin and cephalosporin group" above.

Dosage and Route:

Horses-10,000-40,000 IU/kg, IM, **every 2-3 days**[2]
Cattle-40,000 IU/kg, IM, **every 2-3 days**[2]
Swine-40,000 IU/kg, IM, **every 2-3 days**[2]
Sheep-15,000 IU/kg, IM **every 4-5 days**[1]
Dogs- 40,000 IU/kg, IM, **every 5 days**[2]
Cats-40,000 IU/kg, IM, **every 5 days**[2]
Rabbit-40,000 IU/kg, IM, **every other day**[14]

Withdrawal Period: Note: effective doses greatly exceed the labeled dose, therefore the label withdrawal period must be longer than the label requires.Cattle- IM dosing, meat 21 days, milk 13 days[1] SC dosing, meat 42 days[1]

Precautions: This is a long acting penicillin preparation, take special note of the long time between doses.

PENICILLIN G (procaine)

Indications: See "penicillin and cephalosporin group" above.

Dosage and Route:

Horses- 20,000-50,000 IU/kg, IM, 2-3 times daily[2]
Cattle-20,000-54,000 IU/kg, IM, SC 1-2 times daily[2]
Swine-20,000-54,000 IU/kg, IM, SC 1-2 times daily[2]
Sheep-6-16 mg/kg IM, 1-2 times daily[1]
Llama-40,000 IU/kg, SC, daily[14]
Dogs- 20,000 IU/kg, IM, SC, 1-2 times daily[2]
Cats- 20,000 IU/kg, IM, SC, 1-2 times daily[2]
Rabbit-50,000-100,000 IU/kg, IM, 2 times daily[14]

Withdrawal Period: Note: effective doses greatly exceed the labeled dose, therefore the withdrawal period must be longer than the label specifies.

Cattle- IM dosing, meat 21 days[2] SC dosing, meat 42 days[2]

PENICILLIN V

Indications: See "penicillin and cephalosporin group" above.

Dosage and Route:

Horses- 110,000 IU/kg by mouth, 2-4 times daily[2]; or 42-69 mg/kg by mouth, 3-4 times daily[2]
Dogs- 10 mg/kg, by mouth, 3 times daily[2]
Cats- 10 mg/kg, by mouth, 3 times daily[2]

PEN/STREP (Penicillin G Procaine + Dihydrostreptomycin)

Indications: See "penicillin and cephalosporin group" above. Usually formulated to give 400,000 IU of Pen G Procaine + 0.5 g Dihydrostreptomycin per 2 ml.

Dosage and Route:

Horses- 10-12 ml IM, 1-2 times daily[2]
Foals- 1 ml/22 kg, 1-3 times daily[2]
Cattle-10-12 ml IM, 1-2 times daily[2]
Calves- 1 ml/22 kg, 1-3 times daily[2]
Swine-1 ml/22 kg, 1-3 times daily[2]
Sheep-1 ml/22 kg, 1-3 times daily[2]

Withdrawal Period: Food animals- meat 30 days, milk 3 days[2]

TICARCILLIN

Indications: See "penicillin and cephalosporin group" above.

Dosage and Route:

Horses- 44 mg/kg IM, 3 times daily[3]
Dogs- 55-110 mg/kg SC, IM, IV 3 times daily[3]
Cats- 55-110 mg/kg SC, IM, IV 3 times daily[3]

Aminoglycoside Group

AMIKACIN (Amiglyde, Amikin)

Indications: See "aminoglycoside group" above. Amikacin is a relatively new aminoglycoside antibiotic that is effective against many infections of the genitourinary tract. High cost and prolonged withdrawal period makes amikacin impractical for use in food animals.

Dosage and Route:

Horses- 3.5-7.5 mg/kg SC, IM, 2-4 times daily[2]
Foals- 1-10 mg/kg IM, IV 2 times daily[2]
Cattle-25 mg/kg IM, 2 times daily[3]
Llama-10 mg/kg IM, IV, 2 times daily[14]
Dogs- 5 mg/kg SC,IM, IV 3 times daily[2]
Cats- 5 mg/kg SC,IM, IV 3 times daily[2]

Withdrawal Period: Not normally used in food producing animals due to extremely long time required for residues to diminish. It should only be used to treat life-threatening infections in breeding stock which will not be eaten.

Precautions: Possible kidney damage with high doses for prolonged periods. Do not use in combination with other drugs in the aminoglycoside group.

APRAMYCIN (Apralan)

Indications: See "aminoglycoside group" above. Apramycin is primarily used for oral treatment of scours (diarrhea) in young animals. It is not absorbed from the gut when given orally.

Dosage and Route:

Cattle-20-40 mg/kg by mouth in drinking water[2]
Swine-12.5 mg/kg, by mouth, in drinking water for 7 days
Chicken-500 mg/L in drinking water for 5 days[14]

Withdrawal Period: Swine- meat 28 days

Precautions: Possible kidney damage with high doses for prolonged periods. Do not use in combination with other drugs in the aminoglycoside group.

DIHYDROSTREPTOMYCIN

Note: Dihydrostreptomycin is most commonly available in combination with penicillin G; see Pen/Strep above.

Indications: See "aminoglycoside group" above. Dihydrostreptomycin is the drug of choice for treatment of leptospirosis in cattle.

Dosage and Route:

Horses-11 mg/kg SC, IM, twice daily[2]
Cattle-25 mg/kg IM, daily[2]; or
12.5 mg/kg, IM, twice daily[2]
Dogs- 5-10 mg/kg SC, IM, twice daily[2]; or
12.5 mg/kg SC, IM, 3 times daily[2]
Cats- 5-10 mg/kg SC, IM, twice daily[2]; or
12.5 mg/kg SC, IM, 3 times daily[2]

Withdrawal Period: Cattle- meat 30 days, milk 4 days[2]

Precautions: Possible kidney damage with high doses for prolonged periods. Do not use in combination with other drugs in the aminoglycoside group.

GENTAMICIN (Gentocin, Garamycin)

Indications: See "aminoglycoside group" above. Gentamicin is a readily available and affordable aminoglycide which is commonly given by mouth for scours (diarrhea), by injection for generalized infections, in ophthalmic preparations for treatment of eye infections, and in otic preparations for treatment of ear infections in dogs and cats. Note the prolonged withdrawal periods when injected in cattle and pigs. It is not absorbed from the gut when given orally.

Dosage and Route:

Horses- 2-4 mg/kg, IM, SC, IV, 1 time daily[2]
Cattle-2.2 mg/kg, IM, IV, 3 times daily[2]
Swine-5 mg, IM in 1-3 day old piglets; or
5 mg by mouth in 1-3 day old piglets; or
25 g/gallon of drinking water for 3 days
Llama-2 mg/kg IM, 3 times daily[14]
Dogs- 2 mg/kg, SC, IM, 3 times daily[2]
Cats- 2 mg/kg, SC, IM, 3 times daily[2]
Chicken-0.2-1 mg total dose, SC, 1 time daily[14]
Rabbit-4 mg/kg, IM, 1 time daily[14]
Ferret-5 mg/kg, IM, 1 time daily[14]
Gerbil-5 mg/kg, IM, 1 time daily[14]
Guinea Pig- 5 mg/kg, IM, 1 time daily[14]
Hamster- 5 mg/kg, IM, 1 time daily[14]

Withdrawal:

Cattle-meat 180-360 days, milk 5 days[2]
Swine-if injected, meat 40 days; if oral, meat 3-14 days

Precautions: Possible kidney damage with high doses for prolonged periods. Do not use in combination with other drugs in the aminoglycoside group.

KANAMYCIN

Indications: See "aminoglycoside group" above. Kanamycin is not absorbed from the gut when given orally.

Dosage and Route:

Horses- 7.5 mg/kg IM, IV, 3 times daily[2]
Cattle-6 mg/kg IM, 2 times daily[2]
Swine-6 mg/kg IM, 2 times daily
Dogs- 10-12 mg/kg by mouth, 4 times daily[2]; or
5-7.5 mg/kg SC, IM, 2 times daily[2]
Cats- 10-12 mg/kg by mouth, 4 times daily[2]; or
5-7.5 mg/kg SC, IM, 2 times daily[2]
Rabbit-7 mg/kg IM, SC, 2-4 times daily[14]

Withdrawal Period: Cattle-meat 180-360 days, milk 5 days
Swine-if injected, meat 40 days; if oral, meat 3-14 days

Precautions: Possible kidney damage with high doses for prolonged periods. Do not use in combination with other drugs in the aminoglycoside group.

NEOMYCIN

Indications: See "aminoglycoside group" above. Neomycin is especially toxic to the kidneys when injected. Neomycin is safe when given by mouth and is not absorbed from the gut. It is most commonly used orally to treat bacterial scours (diarrhea).

Dosage and Route:

Horses- Adult 1g/450kg by mouth, 4 times daily; or
2g/450kg by mouth, 2 times daily
Foal 1.5g by mouth, 2 times daily; or
5-15 mg/kg by mouth 1 time daily[3]
Cattle-7-12 mg/kg by mouth, 2 times daily[2]
Swine-7-12 mg/kg by mouth, 2 times daily
Sheep-500 mg by mouth 2 times daily[3]
Goats-500 mg by mouth 2 times daily[3]
Dogs- 2.5-10 mg/kg by mouth, 2-4 times daily; or
3.5 mg/kg SC, IM, IV, 3 times daily[2]
Cats- 2.5-10 mg/kg by mouth, 2-4 times daily; or
3.5 mg/kg SC, IM, IV, 3 times daily[2]
Rabbit-30 mg/kg, by mouth, 2 times daily[14]
Chicken-35-80 mg/L drinking water, or
11 mg/kg by mouth, 1 time daily[14]
Guinea Pig- 8 mg/kg, by mouth, 1 time daily[14]
Hamster-100 mg/kg, SC, 1 time daily[14]

Withdrawal Period: Cattle-meat 30 days, milk 2 days[3]
Swine-meat 20 days[3]
Sheep-meat 20 days[3]

Precautions: Possible kidney damage with high oral doses for prolonged periods or with injection. Do not use in combination with other drugs in the aminoglycoside group.

NETILMICIN

Indications: See "aminoglycoside group" above.

Dosage and Route:

Horses-2 mg/kg IM, IV, 2-3 times daily[2]

Precautions: Possible kidney damage with high doses for prolonged periods. Do not use in combination with other drugs in the aminoglycoside group.

STREPTOMYCIN

Indications: See "aminoglycoside group" above.

Dosage and Route:

Horses-11 mg/kg IM, 2 times daily[5]
Cattle-11 mg/kg IM, 2 times daily[2]
Swine-11 mg/kg IM, 2 times daily
Llama-5 mg/kg, IM, 1 time daily[14]
Dogs- 11-22 mg/kg IM, 2 times daily[2]
Cats- 11-22 mg/kg IM, 2 times daily[2]
Chicken-25-50 mg/kg IM, 1 time daily, or
55 mg/kg by mouth, 1 times daily, or
68-100 mg/L drinking water[14]
Rabbit-60 mg/kg, by mouth daily, or
7-12 mg/kg, IM, 2-3 times daily[14]

Withdrawal Period: Unknown, follow withdrawal for gentamicin injections.

Precautions: Possible kidney damage with high doses for prolonged periods. Do not use in combination with other drugs in the aminoglycoside group.

VANCOMYCIN

Indications: See "aminoglycoside group" above. Vancomycin is not absorbed from the gut when given orally.

Dosage and Route:

Horses- 20-40 mg/kg by mouth or IV, 2-4 times daily[2]

Dogs- 3-15 mg/kg by mouth, 2-4 times daily[2]

Precautions: Possible kidney damage with high doses for prolonged periods. Do not use in combination with other drugs in the aminoglycoside group.

Tetracycline Group

CHLORTRACYCLINE (Aureomycin, Aurofac-D)

Indications: See "tetracycline group" above.

Dosage and Route:

Cattle-10-20 mg/kg by mouth daily[2]
Swine-10-20 mg/kg by mouth daily
Sheep-10-20 mg/kg by mouth daily[1]
Llama-22 mg/kg by mouth daily[14]
Dogs- 25-50 mg/kg by mouth daily[4]
Cats-25-50 mg/kg by mouth daily[4]

Withdrawal Period:

Cattle-meat 10 days[2]
Swine-meat 10 days
Sheep-meat 5 days[1]

Precautions: Do not use in horses. Do not give with milk, or any other antibiotic. It may cause stomach upset.

DOXYCYCLINE

Indications: See "tetracycline group" above.

Dosage and Route:

Dogs- 5-20 mg/kg by mouth, 2 times daily[2]
Cats- 5-20 mg/kg by mouth, 2 times daily[2]

Precautions: Do not use in horses. Do not give with milk, or any other antibiotic. It may cause stomach upset.

OXYTETRACYCLINE (Oxymav, Liquamycin, Terramycin, LA-200, Alamycin)

Indications: See "tetracycline group" above.

Dosage and Route:

Cattle-6-11 mg/kg IM, IV daily; or
10-20 mg/kg by mouth, 4 times daily[2]
Cattle- Long acting injection (LA-200)
20 mg/kg IM once[2]
Swine-6-11 mg/kg IM, IV daily; or
10-20 mg/kg by mouth, 4 times daily[7]
Swine-Long acting injection (LA-200)
20 mg/kg every 2 days[8]
Sheep-10-20 mg/kg by mouth, 4 times daily; or
6-11 mg/kg IM, IV, 1 time daily[3]
Sheep-Long acting injection (LA-200)
20 mg/kg every 3 days[9]
Goats-10-20 mg/kg by mouth, 4 times daily; or
6-11 mg/kg IM, IV, 1 time daily[3]

Goats-Long acting injection (LA-200)
20 mg/kg every 3 days[9]
Llamas-11 mg/kg IV, once daily[14]
Llamas-Long acting injection (LA-200)
20 mg/kg every days[14]
Dogs- 7-12 mg/kg IM, IV 2 times daily; or
22 mg/kg by mouth, 3 times daily[2]
Cats-7-12 mg/kg IM, IV 2 times daily; or
22 mg/kg by mouth, 3 times daily[2]

Withdrawal Period: Cattle by mouth- meat 5 days, milk 4 days[2]
Cattle IM, IV- meat 18 days, milk 3 days[2]
Cattle Long Acting IM- meat 28 days[2]
Swine-Meat 21 days[1]
Sheep-meat 21 days[1]

Precautions: Do not use in horses. Do not give with milk, or any other antibiotics. It may cause stomach upset. If the injection is a large volume divide it into several sites

TETRACYCLINE

Indications: See "tetracycline group" above.

Dosage and Route:
Cattle-5-10 mg/kg by mouth, 2 times daily
Swine-22 mg/kg by mouth in drinking water[3]
Sheep-10 mg/kg by mouth, 2 times daily
Dogs- 25-50 mg/kg by mouth, 3-4 times daily; or
7 mg/kg IM, IV 2 times daily[2]
Cats- 25-50 mg/kg by mouth, 3-4 times daily; or
7 mg/kg IM, IV 2 times daily[2]

Withdrawal Period: Cattle-meat 5 days[2]

Precautions: Do not use in horses. Do not give with milk or any other antibiotic. It may cause stomach upset. If the injection volume is large divide it into several sites

Sulfa Group

SUCCINYLSULFATHIAZOLE

Indications: See "sulfa group" above.

Dosage and Route:

Horses-160 mg/kg by mouth for one day, then 80 mg/kg by mouth daily[5]

Cattle-160 mg/kg by mouth for one day, then 80 mg/kg by mouth daily[5]

Swine-160 mg/kg by mouth for one day, then 80 mg/kg by mouth daily[5]

Sheep-60 mg/kg by mouth for one day, then 80 mg/kg by mouth daily[5]

SULFABROMETHAZINE (Sulfabrom)

Indications: See "sulfa group" above.

Dosage and Route:

Cattle- 130 - 200 mg/kg by mouth[7]

Withdrawal Period: Cattle-10 days, milk 4 days[5]

SULFACHLORPYRIDAZINE (Vetisulid)

Indications: See "sulfa group" above.

Dosage and Route:

Cattle- 65-95 mg/kg by mouth[7]

Swine- 47-75 mg/kg by mouth[7]

Withdrawal Period: Cattle-meat 5 days[6]

SULFADIAZINE

Indications: See "sulfa group" above.

Dosage and Route:

Horses-50 mg/kg by mouth, 2 times daily[5]

Cattle-50 mg/kg by mouth, 2 times daily[5]

Swine-50 mg/kg by mouth, 2 times daily[5]

Sheep-50 mg/kg by mouth, 2 times daily[5]

SULFADIAZINE + TRIMETHOPRIM (Tribrissen)

Indications: See "sulfa group" above.

Dosage and Route:

Horses-30 mg/kg by mouth, 2-3 times daily; or
15 mg/kg IV, 2 times daily[2]
Cattle-30 mg/kg by mouth, one time daily[2]
Swine-48 mg/kg IM daily
Sheep-75 mg/kg by mouth daily[1]; or
13-20 mg/kg IM, SC, IV daily[1]
Dogs-15-30 mg/kg by mouth 1-2 times daily[3]
Cats- 30 mg/kg by mouth 2 times daily[3]

Withdrawal Period: Cattle-meat 3 days, milk 7 days[5]
Swine-meat 10 days
Sheep-meat 14 days[1]

SULFADIMETHOXINE (Bactrovet, Albon)

Indications: See "sulfa group" above.

Dosage and Route:

Horses-25 mg/kg SC, IM, IV for one day, then
12.5 mg/kg SC, IM, IV daily[2]
Cattle- 55 mg/kg by mouth for one day then,
27.5 mg/kg by mouth daily; or
25 mg/kg SC, IM, IV for one day then,
12.5 mg/kg SC, IM, IV daily[2]
Albon SR-137.5 mg/kg every 4 days
Swine-55 mg/kg by mouth for one day then,
27.5 mg/kg by mouth daily[7]
Sheep-55 mg/kg by mouth for one day then,
27.5 mg/kg by mouth daily[5]
Llama-22 mg/kg SC, once daily for 4 days[14]
Dogs- 25 mg/kg by mouth, SC, IM, IV 1-2 times daily[2]
Cats- 25 mg/kg by mouth, SC, IM, IV 1-2 times daily[2]
Chicken-250-500 mg/L drinking water[14]
Rabbit-25 mg/kg by mouth[14]

Withdrawal Period: Cattle-meat 5-7 days, milk 3 days[5]

SULFADIMETHOXINE + ORMETOPRIM (Primor)

Indications: See "sulfa group" above.

Dosage and Route:

Dogs-55 mg/kg by mouth for one day then
27.5 mg/kg by mouth daily[2]

SULFADIMIDINE (Sulfamez)

Indications: See "sulfa group" above.

Dosage and Route:

Cattle- 110 mg/kg by mouth daily[1]; or
150 mg/kg SC daily[1]
Swine- 110 mg/kg by mouth daily[1] 150 mg/kg SC daily[1]
Sheep- 110 mg/kg by mouth daily[1] 215 mg/kg SC daily[1]
Goats- 110 mg/kg by mouth daily[1] 215 mg/kg SC daily[1]

Withdrawal Period: Cattle-meat 15 days, milk 3 days[1]
Swine-meat 15 days[1]
Sheep-meat 15 days[1]
Goats-meat 15 days, milk 3 days[1]

SULFADIMIDINE + TRIMETHOPRIM (Amphoprim, Sulfatrim)

Indications: See "sulfa group" above.

Dosage and Route:

Horses- 13 mg/kg IM, SC, IV daily[1]; or
30 mg/kg by mouth daily[1]
Cattle-13 mg/kg IM, SC, IV daily[1]; or
30 mg/kg by mouth daily[1]
Swine-13 mg/kg IM, SC, IV daily[1]; or
30 mg/kg by mouth daily[1]
Sheep- 13 mg/kg IM, SC, IV daily[1]

Withdrawal Period: Cattle-meat 15 days, milk 3 days[1]
Swine-meat 15 days[1]
Sheep-meat 15 days[1]

SULFADOXINE + TRIMETHOPRIM (Tridox, Trivetrin)

Indications: See "sulfa group" above.

Dosage and Route:

Horse-13-20 mg/kg IV daily[1]
Cattle-13-20 mg/kg IM, IV daily[1]
Swine-13-20 mg/kg IM, IV daily[1]
Sheep-13-20 mg/kg IM, daily[1]
Dogs- 13-20 mg/kg IM, SC, daily[1]
Cats- 13-20 mg/kg IM, SC daily[1]

Withdrawal Period: Cattle-meat 14 days, milk 3 days[1]
Swine-meat 14 days[1]
Sheep-meat 14 days[1]

Precautions: Give by slow IV injection. Do not give IV to cats.

SULFAETHOXYPYRIDAZINE (SEZ)

Indications: See "sulfa group" above.

Dosage and Route:

Cattle-55 mg/kg by mouth daily[5]
Swine-55 mg/kg by mouth daily[5]
Dogs- 20-30 mg/kg by mouth 2 times daily[10]
Cats- 20-30 mg/kg by mouth 2 times daily[10]

Withdrawal Period: Cattle- meat 16 days, milk 3 days[6]

SULFAMETHAZINE

Indications: See "sulfa group" above.

Dosage and Route:

Cattle-200 mg/kg by mouth for one day, then 100 mg/kg one time daily[7]
Swine-200 mg/kg by mouth for one day, then 100 mg/kg one time daily[7]
Sheep-30 ml of 12.5% solution by mouth for one day then 15 ml daily[10]
Dogs- 50 mg/kg by mouth 2 times daily[11]
Cats- 50 mg/kg by mouth 2 times daily[11]
Rabbit-2 g/L drinking water[14]
Chicken-1 g/L drinking water[14]

Withdrawal Period: Cattle-meat 10 days, milk 4 days[5]
Swine-meat 14 days[5]

SULFAMETHOXASOLE + TRIMETHOPRIM (Septra)

Indications: See "sulfa group" above.

Dosage and Route:

Horses-30 mg/kg by mouth, 2-3 times daily; or 15 mg/kg IV 2 times daily[2]
Cattle-30 mg/kg by mouth one time daily[2]
Swine-48 mg/kg IM daily
Llama-45 mg/kg by mouth[14]
Dogs- 15-30 mg/kg by mouth 1-2 times daily[3]
Cats- 30 mg/kg by mouth 2 times daily[3]

SULFA, Triple { 8% sulfamethazine, 8% sulfapyridine & 8% sulfathiazole}

Indications: See "sulfa group" above.

Dosage and Route:

Horses- 41 ml/ 100 lbs IV, then
14 ml/ 100 lbs IV twice daily[10]

Cattle-41 ml/ 100 lbs IV, then
14 ml/ 100 lbs IV twice daily[10]

Swine-41 ml/ 100 lbs IV, then
14 ml/ 100 lbs IV twice daily[10]

Sheep-41 ml/ 100 lbs IV, then
14 ml/ 100 lbs IV twice daily[10]

Withdrawal Period: Cattle-meat 10 days, milk 4 days[5]

SULFAPYRIDINE

Indications: See "sulfa group" above.

Dosage and Route:

Horses-50/mg/kg by mouth daily[4]
Cattle-50/mg/kg by mouth daily[4]
Swine-50/mg/kg by mouth daily[4]
Dogs- 50/mg/kg by mouth daily[4]
Cats- 50/mg/kg by mouth daily[4]

SULFATHIAZOLE

Indications: See "sulfa group" above.

Dosage and Route:

Horses-66 mg/kg by mouth, 3 times daily[5]
Cattle-66 mg/kg by mouth, 6 times daily[5]
Swine-66 mg/kg by mouth, 6 times daily[5]
Sheep-66 mg/kg by mouth, 6 times daily[5]
Chicken-1 g/L drinking water

Miscellaneous Antibiotics

BACITRACIN

Indications: Usually combined with other antibiotics (neomycin and polymixin B) in an ointment or cream for use in the eyes, ears and on external wounds, Bacitracin is too toxic for internal use.

CHLORAMPHENICOL

Indications: Chloramphenicol is a broad spectrum antibiotic that is especially good at penetrating into all tissues of the body. It should not be given with any antibiotics of the penicillin, cephalosporin or aminoglycoside groups. Chloramphenicol is known to produce a fatal blood disease in people, therefore **chloramphenicol should never be used in food producing animals** because residues in the food might cause this fatal reaction in people.

Dosage and Route:

Horses-Chloramphenicol palmitate 25-50 mg/kg by mouth 3-4 times daily (adults)[2]
4-10 mg/kg by mouth 3-4 times daily (foals)[2]
Chloramphenicol succinate 25 mg/kg IM, IV 3-4 times daily[2]

Dogs- 50 mg/kg by mouth, SC, IM, IV 3 times daily[2]

Cats- 50 mg/kg by mouth, SC, IM, IV 2 times daily[2]

Ferret-50 mg/kg by mouth, IM, IV, 2 times daily[14]

Precautions: **Do not use in food producing animals!** Handle with care, do not inhale the powder and wash hands after handling the drug.

CIPROFLOXACIN

Indications: Ciprofloxacin is a very effective antibiotic with good activity against many types of bacteria that cause respiratory and urinary tract infections.

Dosage and Route:

Dogs-2.5- 7.5 mg/kg by mouth, 2 times daily[4]

Cats-2.5- 7.5 mg/kg by mouth, 2 times daily[4]

Rabbits-10-40 mg/kg by mouth, 2 times daily[14]

Precautions: Do not give to young animals as the drug may cause permanent damage to joints.

CLINDAMYCIN (Antirobe)

Indications: Clindamycin is similar to lincomycin. Clindamycin has good activity against many types of bacteria that are resistant to the penicillin group. It is especially good for treatment of wounds, bone infections and abscesses.

Dosage and Route:

Dogs-5-11 mg/kg by mouth, IM, IV, 3 times daily[2]
Cats- 5-11 mg/kg by mouth, IM, IV, 3 times daily[2]

Precautions: Clindamycin may cause fatal reactions in horses, cattle, sheep, goats and rabbits. Do not give with chloramphenicol or erythromycin.

ENROFLOXACIN

Indications: Enrofloxacin is a very effective antibiotic with good activity against many types of bacteria that cause respiratory and urinary tract infections.

Dosage and Route:

Dogs-2.5-7.5 mg/kg by mouth, 2 times daily[4]
Cats-2.5-7.5 mg/kg by mouth, 2 times daily[4]
Chicken-10 mg/kg by mouth, 2 times daily[14]
Ferret-3-10 mg/kg by mouth, IM, SC, 2 times daily[14]
Gerbil-2.5-5 mg/kg by mouth, IM, SC, 2 times daily[14]
Guinea Pig-2.5-5 mg/kg by mouth, IM, SC,2 times daily[14]
Hamster-2.5-5 mg/kg by mouth, IM, SC, 2 times daily[14]
Rabbit-5 mg/kg by mouth, 2 times daily[14]

Precautions: Do not give to young animals as the drug may cause permanent damage to the joints.

ERYTHROMYCIN

Indications: Erythromycin is an antibiotic that is particularly good against gram positive bacteria.

Dosage and Route:

Horses-25 mg/kg by mouth, 3-4 times daily; or
10 mg/kg IM, 2 times daily[3]
Cattle-4-8 mg/kg IM 1-2 times daily[3]
Swine-2.2-6.6 mg/kg IM daily[3];
for young pig scours (diarrhea) give 22 mg/kg IM 1-2 times daily[3]
Sheep-2.2 mg/kg IM daily[3];
for young lamb scours (diarrhea) give 123 mg/kg IM one time[3]
Dogs- 10-20 mg/kg by mouth, 3 times daily[2]

Cats- 10-20 mg/kg by mouth, 3 times daily[2]
Chicken-102 mg/L drinking water[14]
Hamster-20 mg/kg by mouth, 1 time daily[14]
Rabbit-22 mg/kg, IM, 1 time daily[14]

Withdrawal Period: Cattle- meat 14 days, milk 4 days[2]
Swine- meat 7 days[3]
Sheep-meat 3 days[2]

Precautions: Erythromycin may cause vomiting and diarrhea. It may also cause liver problems. Injections often cause swelling and soreness at the site of injection. Do not give with chloramphenicol, lincomycin, clindamycin, kaolin or pectin.

GRISEOFULVIN (Fulvicin)

Indications: Griseofulvin is an oral antibiotic which is only effective against the fungi that cause ringworm. It should be given with a high fat meal to help absorption. People can get ringworm from animals. Everyone who has contact with animals having ringworm should be sure to wash thoroughly after touching the animmals. It is not effective against yeasts like candida.

Dosage and Route:
Horses-10 mg/kg by mouth daily[3]
Cattle-20 mg/kg by mouth daily for 6 weeks[3]
Swine-20 mg/kg by mouth daily for 6 weeks[3]
Sheep-20 mg/kg by mouth daily for 6 weeks[3]
Goats-20 mg/kg by mouth daily for 6 weeks[3]
Llama-10 mg/kg by mouth daily[14]
Dogs- 20-50 mg/kg by mouth daily for 3-6 weeks[2]
Cats- 20-50 mg/kg by mouth dailyfor 3-6 weeks[2]
Rabbit-25 mg/kg by mouth daily for 4-6 weeks[14]

Withdrawal Period: Unknown

Precautions: May cause vomiting or diarrhea. **Do not give to pregnant animals!**

LINCOMYCIN (Lincocin)

Indications: Lincomycin is similar to clindamycin. Lincomycin has good activity against many species of bacteria that are resistant to the penicillin group. It is especially good for treatment of wounds, bone infections and abscesses.

Dosage and Route:

Swine-10 mg/kg, IM daily; or
250 mg/gallon of drinking water[3]
Dogs- 15-25 mg/kg by mouth 2 times daily[3]
Cats- 15-25 mg/kg by mouth 2 times daily[3]
Chicken-17 mg/L drinking water[14]

Withdrawal Period: Swine-meat 6 days

Precautions: Do not give with drugs in the "penicillin group", chloramphenicol or erythromycin. Do not give to horses, cattle, sheep, goats or rabbits. It may cause vomiting and diarrhea in dogs and cats.

NORFLOXACIN

Indications: Norfloxacin is a new type of antibiotic which is too expensive for use in large animals. Norfloxacin is very effective in killing gram positive bacteria, and treating urinary tract, gastrointestinal and respiratory infections.

Dosage and Route:

Dogs-22 mg/kg by mouth, 2 times daily[2]
Cats-22 mg/kg by mouth, 2 times daily[2]

Precautions: Do not give to young animals as the drug may cause permanent damage to joints.

POLYMIXIN B

Indications: Usually combined with other antibiotics (neomycin and bacitracin) in an ointment or cream for use in the eyes, ears and on external wounds. Polymixin B is quite toxic when used internally.

RIFAMPIN

Indications: Rifampin is primarily used to treat the bacteria that cause colitis-X, and pneumonia in young horses. It is also used to treat actinomycosis in dogs and cats.[3] In people it is used to treat tuberculosis.

Dosage and Route:

Horses-2.5-5 mg/kg by mouth, 2 times daily; or
10 mg/kg by mouth, 2 times daily for severe infections[2]
Cattle-2.5-5 mg/kg by mouth[2]
Dogs- 10-20 mg/kg by mouth, 2 times daily[2]
Cats- 10-20 mg/kg by mouth, 2 times daily[2]

Precautions: Rifampin stains urine, tears, saliva and sweat reddish orange. It may cause vomiting, diarrhea and rashes.[3]

SPECTINOMYCIN

Indications: Spectinomycin is similar in action to the 'Aminoglycoside group" of antibiotics and has good activity against gut bacteria. It primarily used in swine to control scours but is occasionally used to treat pneumonia and scours in other animals. When given by mouth it is not absorbed.[3]

Dosage and Route:

Horses-20 mg/kg IM, 3 times daily[3]
Cattle-12 mg/kg IM, daily[2]
Swine- 10 mg/kg by mouth, IM, 2 times daily[3]
Dogs- 5-12 mg/kg IM, 2 times daily; or
20 mg/kg by mouth, 2 times daily[2]
Cats-5-12 mg/kg IM, 2 times daily ; or
20 mg/kg by mouth, 2 times daily[2]
Chicken-135-530 mg/L drinking water[14]

Withdrawal Period: Cattle-meat 30 days, milk 4 days[2]
Swine-meat 21 days[3]

Precautions: Spectinomycin may cause soreness at the injection site. Do not use with chloramphenicol or tetracycline.

SPIRAMYCIN (Stomorgyl)

Indications: Spiramycin is an antibiotic that is particularly good against gram positive bacteria and for the treatment of swine dysentery.

Dosage and Route:

Dogs-75,000 IU/kg by mouth daily[1]
Cats- 75,000 IU/kg by mouth daily[1]
Chicken-400 mg/L drinking water[14]

Precautions: Spiramycin may cause vomiting and diarrhea. It may also cause liver problems. Do not give with chloramphenicol, lincomycin, clindamycin, kaolin or pectin.

TIAMULIN (Denagard)

Indications: Tiamulin is only used to treat pneumonia and dysentery of swine.

Dosage and Route:

Swine-dysentery- 7.7 mg/kg by mouth indrinking water for 5 days[3]
pneumonia- 223.1 mg/kg by mouth in drinking water for 5 days[3]

Withdrawal Period: Swine-3 days for low dose[3] 7 days for high dose[3]

Precautions: The skin may become red during this treatment. Toxic doses may cause vomiting and salivation.[3]

TILMICOSIN PHOSPHATE (Micotil 300)

Indications: Tilmicosin is a new long-acting antibiotic that is primarily used to treat shipping fever (bacterial and viral) pneumonia in cattle. Do not use in cattle producing milk for human consumption.[2]

Dosage and Route:

Cattle-10 mg/kg SC, once[2]

Withdrawal Period: Cattle- meat 28 days, milk do not use[2]

Precautions: Intravenous injection in cattle, and any use in swine has been fatal. Avoid contact with the eyes. Do not inject more than 25 ml in any one site. Injection sites may be sore.

TYLOSIN (Tylan)

Indications: Tylosin is a broad spectrum antibiotic that is most commonly used to treat swine dysentery and diarrhea in other animals.

Dosage and Route:

Cattle-17.6 mg/kg IM, daily[2]
Swine-8.8 mg/kg IM, 2 times daily; 5-10 mg/kg by mouth
Sheep-10 mg/kg by mouth for 5 days;[3] or
400 mg IM, daily for 2 days for Chlamydial abortion
Goats-10 mg/kg by mouth for 5 days; or
6.6 mg/kg IM, daily
Dogs- 5-10 mg/kg by mouth, 2-3 times daily; or
5-15 mg/kg IM, IV, 3-4 times daily[2]
Cats-5-10 mg/kg by mouth, 2-3 times daily; or
5-15 mg/kg IM, IV, 3-4 times daily[2]
Ferret-10 mg/kg by mouth, 3 times daily, or
5-10 mg/kg IM, IV, 2 times daily[14]
Gerbil-10 mg/kg by mouth, IM, SC, 1 time daily[14]
Guinea Pig-10 mg/kg by mouth, IM, SC, 1 time daily[14]
Hamster-10 mg/kg, IM, SC, 1 time daily[14]
Chicken-530 mg/L drinking water[14]
Rabbit-5-10 mg/kg by mouth, IM, SC, 1-2 times daily[14]

Withdrawal Period: Cattle-meat 21 days, milk do not use[2]
Swine-meat 14 days[3]

Precautions: Tylosin can kill horses. Do not use in cattle producing milk for human consumption. Tylosin may cause loss of appetite, diarrhea or pain at the injection site. Do not inject more than 5 ml per site.

ANTI-INFLAMMATORY DRUGS

Inflammation is the body's response to microbial, chemical or physical injury. Inflammation causes heat (fever), redness, pain, swelling and loss of function. A good example of this process is a bee sting. In most cases inflammation is the body's way of fighting the attack, controlling damage and beginning the process of repair. In some cases the inflammatory process can become a long term problem. In these cases it may be helpful to decrease the inflammation by giving anti-inflammatory drugs. These drugs come in two large groups "steroids" and "non-steroids." "Steroids" resemble hormones made in the body like cortisone that normally limit inflammation. "Non steroids" are synthetic drugs like aspirin that block the signs of inflammation. Each group has its own set of good and bad effects. "Steroids" decrease the body's defense against infectious disease and produce excessive appetite, weight gain, water consumption and urination. "Non-steroids" can irritate and cause ulceration of the gastrointestinal tract. Animals are typically more sensitive to the gastrointestinal side effects of non-steroids than people. The following list of anti-inflammatory drugs includes those that are most commonly available for use in animals.

"Steroids"

DEXAMETHASONE

Indications: Dexamthasone is a potent and long lasting steroid anti-inflammatory. It is useful in the treatment of arthritis, lameness, and muscular injuries.

Dosage and Route:

Horses-0.02-0.2 mg/kg by mouth, IM, IV, daily[2]
Cattle-5-10 mg/kg IM, IV, daily[2]
Swine-1-10 mg IM, IV, daily[3]
Dogs-0.25-1.25 mg by mouth, daily for 3-5 days; or[3]
0.5-1 mg IM, IV, daily for 3-5 days[3]
Cats-0.125-0.5 by mouth, IM, IV, daily, for 3-5 days[3]
Rabbit-2.6-4 mg/kg IM, as needed[14]

Withdrawal Period: Unknown

Precautions: Dexamethasone can induce labor and abortion in pregnant animals. It can induce laminitis (founder) in horses. It should not be used in animals that have bacterial, viral or fungal disease due to its effect of decreasing the immune response. Do not use with any other steroid or non-steroid anti-inflammatory drugs.

PREDNISONE

Indications: Prednisone is a medium duration steroid that is useful in the treatment of arthritis, lameness, and muscular injuries. It is almost identical to prednisolone.

Dosage and Route:

Horses-0.25-1.0 mg/kg IM daily[3]
Cattle-0.2-1.0 mg/kg IM daily[3]
Swine-0.2-1.0 mg/kg IM daily[3]
Llama-2 mg/kg by mouth daily[14]
Dogs- 0.5 mg/kg by mouth, every 1-2 days[3]
Cats- 1-2 mg/kg by mouth, every 1-2 days[3]

Precautions: Prednisone can induce labor and abortion in pregnant animals. It can induce laminitis (founder) in horses. It should not be used in animals that have bacterial, viral or fungal disease due to its effect of decreasing the immune response. Do not use with any other steroid or non-steroid anti-inflammatory drugs.

PREDNISOLONE

Indications: Prednisolone is a medium duration steroid that is useful in the treatment of arthritis, lameness, and muscular injuries. It is almost identical to prednisone.

Dosage and Route:

Horses-0.25-1.0 mg/kg IM daily[3]
Cattle-0.2-1.0 mg/kg IM daily[3]
Swine-0.2-1.0 mg/kg IM daily[3]
Dogs- 0.5 mg/kg by mouth, every 1-2 days[3]
Cats- 1-2 mg/kg by mouth, every 1-2 days[3]

Withdrawal Period: Unknown.

Precautions: Prednisolone can induce labor and abortion in pregnant animals. It can induce laminitis (founder) in horses. It should not be used in animals that have bacterial, viral or fungal disease due to its effect of decreasing the immune response. Do not use with any other steroid or non-steroid anti-inflammatory drugs.

Non-steroids

ASPIRIN

Indications: Aspirin is a non-steroid anti-inflammatory drug that has three main effects, it fights inflammation, fever and pain. See also page XXX.

Dosage and Route:

Horses-15-100 mg/kg by mouth, 2-3 times daily[2]
Cattle-15-100 mg/kg by mouth, 2-3 times daily[2]
Swine-10 mg/kg by mouth, 4 times daily[3]
Dogs- 10 mg/kg by mouth, 2 times daily for fever[2]; or 25-35 mg/kg by mouth, 3 times daily for pain[2]
Cats- 6 mg/kg by mouth, **every 2-3 days** for fever[2]; or 10 mg/kg by mouth, **every 2 days** for pain[2]

Precautions: Aspirin can cause stomach upset and ulcers it is best to give with a meal. At very high doses it can cause sickness and death. Use with great caution in cats. Do not use in pregnant animals. **Keep away from children!**

DMSO (Dimethylsulfoxide, Domoso)

Indications: DMSO is potent solvent that penetrates all tissues (including those of the person who applies it!). It reduces pain, inflammation and is very effective in treating sore joints. DMSO is virtually non-toxic. See also page XXX.

Dosage and Route:

Horses-apply to painful area 2 times daily[2]
Cattle-apply to painful area 2 times daily[2]
Swine-apply to painful area 2 times daily
Dogs- apply to painful area 2 times daily[2]
Cats- apply to painful area 2 times daily[2]

Withdrawal Period: Cattle-meat 20 days. milk 3 days[2]

Precautions: Wear gloves when applying to the animal, if gloves are not available then wash hands thoroughly after application. It produces an unusual oyster-like taste in the mouth, and a garlic-like breath when it has been absorbed. Do not use for more than 30 days in horses.

FLUNIXIN MEGLUMINE (Banamine, Finadyne)

Indications: Flunixin meglumine is a very potent (aspirin-like) anti-inflammatory which is used primarily in horses and cattle to treat lameness, colic, and calf scours (diarrhea).

Dosage and Route:

Horses-1.1 mg/kg by mouth, IM, IV, 1-3 times daily[2]
Cattle-2.2 mg/kg IV every 12 hours if needed for a total of 3 doses[2]
Swine-2.2 mg/kg by deep IM injection every 12 hours if needed for a total of 3 doses (according to Australian Package insert)
Llama-0.5-1 mg/kg IV 1-2 times daily[14]
Dogs-0.5-1.0 mg/kg IV only once or twice[2]

Withdrawal Period: Cattle-meat 14 days, milk 4 days[2]

Precautions: Do not use in cats. Use with caution in pregnant animals. High doses for prolonged periods **will cause** gastrointestinal ulcers. The drug relieves pain so well that it has also been accused of masking the severity of colic and therefore delaying more effective treatment like surgery. Do not use in combination with any other anti-inflammatory drugs.

PHENYLBUTASONE (Bute, Butazolidin)

Indications: Phenylbutasone is a potent (aspirin-like) anti-inflammatory drug that has been used successfully for many years. It has three main effects, it fights inflammation, fever and pain. It is not effective in treating the pain of colic. Several days of treatment may be needed to see the full effect of the drug. See also page 221.

Dosage and Route:

Horses-2-4.4 mg/kg by mouth, 1-2 times daily[2]
Cattle-4-8 mg/kg by mouth; or
2-5 mg/kg IV every 2 days[2]
Swine-4-8 mg/kg by mouth daily; or
2-5 mg/kg IV[3]
Llama-2-4 mg/kg by mouth daily[14]
Dogs- 14 mg/kg by mouth, 3 times daily
maximum dose 800 mg/day[2]

Withdrawal Period: Cattle-meat 14 days, milk 5 days[2]

Precautions: High doses and prolonged administration can cause loss of appetite, ulcers in the mouth and mouth. Severe toxicity can cause death. Do not use in cats.

VITAMINS & MINERALS

Nutritional insufficiency is common in developing countries due to short supplies of affordable high quality feedstuffs and overwhelming parasite infections. Vitamin and mineral deficiencies are especially common. Animals that are deficient in these micro nutrients are more likely to be sick and less likely to recover and heal. When treating any animal in a developing country, the nutritional status should be considered. If the animal is well nourished, then compliment the owner on their good work. If the animal is undernourished, evaluate the feeding program and feedstuffs available. Treat the vitamin and mineral needs and counsel the owner in how to improve the nutrition of their animals. The other books in the CVM series are an excellent resource to understanding the nutritional needs and proper feeding of animals in developing countries.

IRON DEXTRAN

Indications: Iron dextran is iron complexed with a dextran molecule to allow slow release of the iron. This complex is necessary because too much iron can be toxic and fatal. Calculate the dose carefully and keep away from children. Iron dextran is most often needed for growing pigs prior to weaning. It may also be needed for animals that have lost a large amount of blood from an injury, or from severe parasite infestations.

Dosage and Route:

Horses-500-1,000 mg IM (split into 2-3 sites) every 7 days[1]

Swine-100-200 mg IM, 1-4 day old pigs; or 50-100 mg IM, every 7 days[1]

Dogs- 10-20 mg IM once[2]

Cats- 50 mg IM once[2]

Withdrawal Period: None required

Precautions: Iron can be toxic and fatal. Calculate the dose carefully and keep away from children. Injection into pigs over 28 days old may cause staining of the muscle.

VITAMIN A & D INJECTION

Indications: Vitamins A & D are fat soluble vitamins, often deficient when feed quality is lacking. The concentration and directions for use may vary from country to country. The doses listed are a guide for the U.S. products which contain 500,000 IU vitamin A and 75,000 IU vitamin D3 per ml.

Dosage and Route:

Cattle- Adult 2-4 ml IM[12]
Yearlings 1-2 ml IM[12]
Calves 0.5 - 1.0 ml IM[12]

Swine- Adult 1-2 ml IM[12]
Growing 0.5 - 1.0 ml IM[12]
Baby Pigs 0.25-0.5 ml IM

Sheep- Adult 1-2 ml IM[12]
Fattening Lambs 0.5-1.0 ml IM[12]
Lambs 0.25-.05 ml IM[12]

Note: they can also be given orally, follow the label directions, do not exceed label directions, these vitamins can be toxic if given too long.

Withdrawal Period: Meat 60 days[12]

Precautions: The injection can be quite painful, make certain the animal is properly restrained.

VITAMIN B-COMPLEX INJECTION

Indications: The B-complex vitamins are an assortment of closely related water soluble vitamins including: thiamine (B1), Riboflavin (B2), niacin, panthenol, pyridoxine (B6), inositol, and choline. The concentration and directions may vary from country to country. The doses listed are a guide.

Dosage and Route:

Horses-1-5 ml/50 kg, IM, IV[12]
Cattle-1-5 ml/50 kg, IM, IV[12]
Swine-1-5 ml/50 kg, IM, IV[12]
Sheep-1-5 ml/50 kg, IM, IV[12]

Note: they can also be given orally, follow the label directions.

Withdrawal Period: None required

Precautions: Protect from light, sunlight and heat which can destroy these vitamins. The products may stain if spilled on skin or clothing. The injection can be quite painful, make certain the animal is properly restrained.

ANTIDOTES

ATROPINE

Indications: Atropine is used as an antidote for organophosphate insecticide poisoning. Doses listed are a guide. Atropine should be given in high enough doses and often enough to control he signs of organophosphate poisoning.

Dosage and Route:

Horses-0.22 mg/kg IM, SC[3]
Cattle-0.5 mg/kg IM, SC
Swine-0.22 mg/kg IM, SC[3]
Sheep-0.5 mg/kg IM, SC[3]
Goats-0.5 mg/kg IM, SC[3]
Dogs-0.2-2.0 mg/kg IM, SC[3]
Cats-0.2-2.0 mg/kg IM, SC[3]

Withdrawal Period: not known

Precautions: Atropine should be used with caution in horses, as it may stop normal intestinal movements (ileus). High doses can cause excitement, dry mouth, vomiting, constipation, seizures, rapid heart rate and shock.

CHARCOAL, ACTIVATED

Indications: Activated charcoal is used to treat poisoning. It adsorbs and binds to poisons in the gastrointestinal tract and prevent them from getting into the animals' system.

Dosage and Route: Prepare the charcoal in enough water to form a slurry and give by mouth or tube.

Horses- Foal 250 grams[3]
Adult 500-750 grams[3]
Cattle-1-3 grams/kg[3]
Sheep-1-3 grams/kg[3]
Goats-1-3 grams/kg[3]
Dogs-2 grams/kg[3]
Cats-2 grams/kg[3]

Withdrawal Period: unknown

Precautions: Activated charcoal can cause vomiting, constipation or diarrhea. Activated charcoal should not be used in cases of poisoning by strong acids, bases or petroleum products.[3]

EPINEPHRINE (Adrenaline)

Indications: Epinephrine is used as an emergency drug to treat anaphylaxis. Anaphylaxis is a severe, sudden, life threatening allergic reaction brought on by insect sting, vaccination or exposure to penicillin.

Dosage and Route: For the 1:1,000 solution (1 mg/ml)

Horses- 0.3-0.5 ml per 45 kg IM, SC
Cattle-0.5-1.0 ml per 45 kg IM, SC[3]
Swine-0.5-1.0 ml per 45 kg IM, SC[3]
Sheep-0.5-1.0 ml per 45 kg IM, SC[3]
Goats-0.5-1.0 ml per 45 kg IM, SC[3]
Dogs-0.1-0.2 ml per 10 kg IV, IM, SC[3]
Cats-0.1 ml IV, SC[3]

(For the 1:10,000 solution give 10 times the volume listed above because it contains 0.1 mg/ml)

Precautions: Epinephrine can cause fear, excitement, vomiting, increased heart rate and irregular heart rate. The effects of epinephrine only last for a few minutes but usually the dose does not need to be repeated.

Antidiarrhea Drugs

BISMUTH SUBSALICYLATE (Pepto-Bismol)

Indications: Bismuth subsalicylate is an oral drug used in people and animals to treat stomach upset and diarrhea. It protects the gut by adsorbing bacteria and toxins and decreases the secretion of water into the gut, decreasing the volume of fluid lost into the gut.

Dosage and Route:

Horses-0.5 ml/kg by mouth, 4-6 times daily[3]
Calves-60 ml by mouth, 2-4 times daily[3]
Baby Pigs- 2-5 ml by mouth, 2-4 times daily[3]
Dogs-2 ml/kg by mouth, 3-4 times daily[3]

Precautions: Do not use in cats, because the salicylate may be toxic. Do not use in animals with bleeding ulcers.

KAOLIN/PECTIN (Kaopectate)

Indications: Kaolin/Pectin is a mixture of kaolin which is a refined type of clay, and pectin which is obtained from apples or citrus fruit. It is used to treat the clinical signs associated with diarrhea. It is thought to bind bacterial toxins, coat the gut and improve the consistency of feces.

Dosage and Route:

Horses- Adult 2-4 liters by mouth, twice daily[3]
Foal 90-120 ml by mouth, 3-4 times daily[3]
Cattle-Adult120-300 ml by mouth, 6-12 times daily[3]
Calves 60-90 ml by mouth, 6-12 timesdaily[3]
Pigs-15-60 ml by mouth, 6-12 times daily[3]
Sheep-90-120 ml by mouth, 6-8 times daily[3]
Dogs-1-2 ml/kg by mouth, 4-12 times daily[3]
Cats-1-2 ml/kg by mouth, 4-12 times daily[3]

Precautions: Prolonged therapy with high doses may cause constipation or impaction. Discontinue therapy as soon as possible.

Other Drugs

MAGNESIUM HYDROXIDE (Milk of Magnesia)

Indications: Magnesium hydroxide is a laxative.

Dosage and Route:

Horses-200-250 ml by mouth, 3 times daily[2]
Cattle-100-454 g in water slurry by mouth[2]
Swine-3-30 ml/kg by mouth[7]
Sheep-50-100 g in water slurry by mouth
Dogs-15-150 ml by mouth, 1-2 times daily[2]
Cats-15-150 ml by mouth, 1-2 times daily[2]

Precautions: Prolonged therapy with high doses can produce diarrhea.

MAGNESIUM SULFATE (Epsom Salts)

Indications: Magnesium sulfate is an oral laxative.

Dosage and Route:

Horses-0.2-0.4 g/kg dissolved in warm water, given by mouth, once daily[2]
Cattle-1-2 g/kg dissolved in warm water, given by mouth, once daily[2]
Swine-1-2 g/kg dissolved in warm water, given by mouth[3]
Sheep-1-2 g/kg dissolved in warm water, given by mouth[3,10]
Dogs- 2-60 g dissolved in warm water, given by mouth[3]
Cats-2-5 g dissolved in warm water, given by mouth[3]

Precautions: Prolonged therapy with high doses of magnesium sulfate can produce diarrhea.

MINERAL OIL

Indications: Mineral oil is also known as white petrolatum, liquid petrolatum, liquid paraffin and white mineral oil. It Is a tasteless, odorless, transparent, colorless, oily liquid that is insoluble in water. It is most commonly used in horses to treat constipation, and fecal impaction and is also used as a laxative in other species. **It must be given by stomach tube to prevent aspiration into the lungs and foreign body pneumonia.**

Dosage and Route:

Horses-2-4 liters by stomach tube[3]
Cattle-1-4 liters by stomach tube[3]
Swine-50-100 ml by stomach tube[3]
Sheep-100-500 ml by stomach tube[3]
Goats-100-500 ml by stomach tube[3]
Dogs-2-60 mls by stomach tube[3]
Cats-2-10 mls by stomach tube[3]

Precautions: Mineral oil must be given by stomach tube to prevent aspiration into the lungs and foreign body pneumonia.

Antiseptics and Disinfectants

An antiseptic is an agent that prevents infection by inhibiting the growth of germs. These agents are safe for use on living tissue, to treat cuts, wounds and sores. A disinfectant is an agent that is used to inhibit the growth of germs on non-living objects, like scalpels, needles, boots and other equipment. Sometimes the same chemical can be used as both an antiseptic and disinfectant, using strong solutions to clean the skin in preparation for surgery (surgical prep) or for disinfecting medical equipment, and using diluted solutions on open wounds. Wounds and equipment should be washed clean of dirt, body fluids or debris for proper disinfection/antisepsis to occur. See the appendix for instructions on dilution.

ALCOHOL

Indications: Alcohols like isopropyl "rubbing alcohol" (50-70%) or ethanol "grain or denatured alcohol" (70%) are sometimes used to kill bacteria. The alcohols take some time to kill bacteria but do not kill bacteria spores, or fungi. They may be used on skin or equipment, but should not be used in open wounds. They are not very good at disinfecting equipment.

Dosage and Route: Use full strength on intact skin and equipment.

Precautions: Do not use on open wounds. Very flammable. Denatured alcohol and rubbing alcohol are poisonous if ingested. Make certain that these alcohols are not available to people who are likely to abuse alcohol.

CHLORHEXIDINE (Nolvasan, Virosan)

Indications: Chlorhexidine is one of the safest and most effective antiseptics available. It has very good activity against bacteria, molds, yeasts and viruses. It works rapidly. It is available as a plain solution, and as a scrub solution. The scrub solution contains a detergent and should be rinsed off after use. The plain solution is very good at rinsing and soaking open wounds.

Dosage and Route:

Surgical Prep-2.0-4.0%[13]
Open Wounds- 0.05%[13]
Disinfection-0.5-2.0%[13]

Precautions: Do not use the strong solutions on open wounds. The solution may form a precipitate in storage, but this does not affect its' usefulness. It is incompatible with hard water and some detergents.

CHLORINE BLEACH (Sodium Hypochlorite)

Indications: Chlorine bleach is readily available and is particularly effective in killing viruses and bacteria. It can be used full strength for disinfection or diluted for use in wounds, but it can damage living tissues.[13]

Dosage and Route:

Open wounds- 0.125% (1/4 strength)

Disinfection-0.5% (full strength)

Precautions: Do not use on living tissue if better agents are available. Be careful when handling the solution because it is a powerful oxidizer and will bleach fabrics and other materials. Do not mix with ammonia or any other cleaning or disinfection agents, as toxic fumes may result.

COPPER NAPHTHENATE (Kopertox, Cuperi-nox)

Indications: Copper naphthenate is a preparation that is used to treat foot rot and thrush in the feet of livestock. It has antiseptic and caustic qualities.

Dosage and Route: Clean affected feet thoroughly and apply full strength. Do not apply to skin.

Precautions: Do not allow copper naphthenate to get onto skin as it will cause hair loss. Do not contaminate feed.

CRESOL

Indications: Cresol compounds effective in killing bacteria but have less effect on bacterial spores, viruses or fungi. They are primarily used to disinfect non-living surfaces.

Dosage and route: Use as directed to clean and disinfect non-living surfaces.

Precautions: Cresol imparts a foul odor to the premises. Do not use or store around human food. It is poisonous and should be handled carefully.

FORMALDEHYDE

Indications: Formaldehyde is a very potent solution which is extremely effective in killing germs on non-living surfaces.

Dosage: Use as a disinfectant on non-living surfaces.

Precautions: Formaldehyde should only be used where adequate ventilation is available. It is quite toxic when confined in a small space. It is corrosive to metal.

FURAZOLIDONE
NITROFURADONE

Indications: Furazolidone (Furoxone) and nitrofuradone (Furacin) are nitrofurans that are effective in inhibiting the growth of bacteria. The are available as powders, ointments, and sprays that are used directly on wounds.

Dosage and Route: Use directly on open wounds as directed on the label. Special preparations are used to treat pinkeye in cattle.

Precautions: Clean the wound before beginning therapy with these products.

HYDROGEN PEROXIDE

Indications: Hydrogen peroxide is a readily available solution usually prepared in a 3% solution. It readily foams and hisses when poured into an open wound. Hydrogen peroxide is very good at flushing out abscesses because it releases oxygen into the wound which is toxic to bacteria. It is also toxic to animal tissues and should only be used for initial cleaning and flushing of dirty wounds and abscesses. Repeated use may retard healing.

Dosage and Route: Use full strength 3% solution on wounds and abcesses.[13]

Precautions: Toxic to animal tissues and should only be used for initial cleaning and flushing of dirty wounds and abscesses. Repeated use may retard healing.

IODINE

Indications: The standard "drug store" iodine tincture is a 2% solution that is painted directly on small cuts and scrapes. A stronger 7% iodine is sometimes used in veterinary medicine as a caustic and is used to treat the umbilical cords of newborn livestock.

Dosage and route: Small cuts and scratches- 2% iodine
Umbilical cords-7% iodine

Precautions: Do not confuse the two different iodine solutions. The 7% solution is caustic and should not be used on burns and deep wounds. Keep both solutions away from eyes, and away from flames.

PHENOL

Indications: Phenol compounds (carbolic acid, Listerine & Lysol) are very effective in killing bacteria but have less effect on bacterial spores, viruses or fungi. They are primarily used to disinfect non-living surfaces.

Dosage and route: Use as directed to clean and disinfect non-living surfaces.

Precautions: Phenol imparts a foul odor to the premises, it should not be used around human food.

POVIDONE-IODINE (Betadine)

Indications: Povidone-iodine (tamed iodine) is one of the safest and most effective antiseptics available. It has very good activity against bacteria, molds, yeasts and viruses and works rapidly. It is available as a plain solution, and as a scrub solution. The scrub solution has a detergent in it which should be rinsed off after use. The plain solution is very good at rinsing and soaking open wounds.

Dosage and Route: Surgical Prep-7.5% preparation[13]
Open Wounds-0.1-1.0% preparation[13]

Precautions: Do not use the strong solutions on open wounds. The solution is corrosive to metals.

PURPLE WOUND SPRAY

Indications: "Purple Wound Spray" is a common veterinary preparation in the United States. It contains isopropyl alcohol, methyl violet, and tannic acid in an aerosol spray can. It has some antibacterial and astringent activity.

Dosage and Route: Apply as directed to minor scrapes and wounds of livestock.

Precautions: Keep away from flame when applying.

QUATERNARY AMMONIUM

Indications: Quaternary ammonium compounds like benzalkonium chloride (Roccal) can be used for disinfection and in diluted form on wounds. It is not normally used on wounds due to availability of better and safer agents.

Dosage: Use as directed as a disinfectant for non-living surfaces

Precautions: In concentrated solutions it is irritating and can cause burns.

ZINC OXIDE OINTMENT

Indications: Zinc oxide ointment has some mild antibacterial activity. It can be used to treat minor cuts and scrapes.

Dosage and Route: Apply as needed to minor cuts and scrapes 2-3 times daily.

Precautions: None

SECTION 8

VACCINES

VIII. VACCINES

THE IMMUNE SYSTEM

The immune system is the body's major defense against invasion by foreign proteins and microorganisms. This defense mechanism is highly complex and not totally understood.

In very general terms, each animal has a permanent record of the make-up of the cells of its own body. This permanent record prevents the body's immune system from attacking its own cells and tissues. When a substance enters the body through the skin, mouth (gut), nose or mucous membrane certain cells recognize it as foreign. A template is made of all or part of the foreigner for future recognition and the immune system attempts to remove the foreigner from the body. The defense cells react best to protein or a partial protein foreigner, whereas objects like B-B gunshot cause little defense reaction in the body.

Some of the defense cells will produce antibodies which are protein molecules which bind to foreign invaders and help kill them. Some of these defense cells will make a permanent record (memory) of the foreigner so that the body can quickly produce antibodies against the invader if needed in the future.

Immunoprophylaxis

Immunoprophylaxis can be defined as the promotion of a specific immune response in an animal in an attempt to protect it against infectious disease. This can be done actively through vaccines containing microorganisms or parts of microorganisms or chemicals produced by microorganisms. This can also be done passively through the transfer of factors (antibodies) obtained from another animal.

Passive Immunization

Passive transfer of antibodies from the mother to her offspring occurs primarily through the colostrum (the first milk). The protection transferred to the neonate depends on the dam's antibody level and the quantity of colostrum received during nursing. In general, nursing must occur within the first 72 hours of the neonate's life in order for colostrum to be adequately absorbed from the gastrointestinal tract. After this point the uptake of antibodies from the gut stops. The amount of antibody in the dam's colostrum is directly related to her immune status for each disease. Therefore, previous exposure and vaccination status directly affect the colostrum antibody level. Usually pregnant animals should be vaccinated 30 days prior to giving birth to enhance the dam's protection and the production of colostral antibodies.

The protection given to the neonate from passive transfer usually lasts from 6 to 12 weeks. This protection will interfere with attempts to provide active immunity through vaccination. Once the maternal antibodies are gone from the young, then immunization must be given to provide immunity against disease.

Passive immunization can be accomplished through the administration of antisera. Antiserum can be used to prevent disease or to treat disease. Examples of diseases in which antisera are used are tetanus and neonatal calf scours caused by *E. coli.* The efficacy of passive immunization depends on many factors. The quantity of antibody given must be great enough to fight the disease. Some diseases are not curable simply by an antibody defense. Timing between exposure to the microorganisms and the administration of the antisera is critical. Perhaps the disease process has gone too far. Depending on the product used and the species to which it is given, allergic reactions and transfer of another infectious agent is possible. The duration of immunity provided by antiserum is short lived.

Active Immunization

Active immunization results from administration of a vaccine against a specific disease causing agent. The vaccine must cause the body to mount an immune response which makes it resistant to the agent. Vaccines must be thoroughly researched to insure safety and efficacy. A vaccine's performance in an animal is affected by conditions such as stress, nutrition, concurrent disease, parasitism, other medications given, individual variation and reduced immunologic competency.

There are four basic types of vaccines classified according to the form of microorganism used -- live, modified live, killed, and subunit (specific pieces of the organism). The following chart lists the advantages, disadvantages, and indications of use for each type.

MODIFIED LIVE VACCINE (ATTENUATED VACCINE)

Advantages

- Rapid protection
- Long protection
- Fewer microorganisms needed

- Reproduction of the microorganism simulates natural infection process which stimulates multiple protective immune pathways

Disadvantages

- Risk of contamination with other infectious agents
- Must be stored and handled correctly to prevent damage to vaccine
- Requires more testing to insure safety and potency prior to release for sale
- Requires reproduction in animal to be effective
- The agent might change back into disease causing form

Indications

- Routine vaccination
- Vaccination in the midst of an outbreak

KILLED VACCINE (INACTIVATED VACCINE)

Advantages

- The agent cannot return to disease causing form
- More stable in storage

Disadvantages

- Minimum of 2 doses for best protection
- More risk of allergic reaction
- Shorter immunity
- More microorganisms needed
- Adjuvant is commonly added to insure adequate stimulation to the animal's immune system

Indications

- Pregnant animals
- Debilitated animals
- Neonates who did not nurse colostrum

SUBUNIT VACCINE

Advantages

- Minimal foreign protein therefore less allergic reactions
- Can be highly potent

Disadvantage

- Expensive to develop and manufacture

Indications

- Pregnant animals
- Debilitated animals

LIVE VACCINE (controlled numbers of disease producing microorganisms) Live vaccines are made with the disease producing microorganisms. The theory is to give enough live organisms to stimulate a good immune response but not enough to cause disease. As one might imagine this balance can be a problem to achieve.

GENERAL GUIDELINES FOR VACCINE ADMINISTRATION

* The withdrawal period is usually 21 days, but some require 60 days. CHECK THE LABEL.
* DO NOT chemically disinfect syringes and needles used to administer vaccines. Chemical residue could render the vaccine ineffective.
* Vaccinate pregnant animals 2-4 weeks prior to expected birthing.
* Do not give antisera and vaccines at the same time. The antisera may block the vaccine from working.
* Vaccinate only healthy animals.
* READ THE LABEL INSTRUCTIONS COMPLETELY PRIOR TO USE.

AVIAN VACCINES

Information for avian vaccines was compounded from Compendium of Veterinary Products, K. Bennett, B.S., 1993.

FORMAT AND ABBREVIATIONS

Name of microorganism and/or names of associated diseases:

Vaccine Type:	L	- live vaccine
	K	- killed vaccine
	ML	- modified live vaccine
	SU	- subunit vaccine
	MV	- monovalent (microorganism is the only one in vaccine)
	C	- Compound (multiple microorganisms are In vaccine)
Information:	WD	- withdrawal period

ADENOVIRUS (Hemorrhagic enteritis of turkeys)

Vaccine Type: ML. MV

Information: For turkeys vaccinate turkeys beginning at 4 to 6 weeks of age depending on the vaccine used. WD-21 days for slaughter.

BORDATELLA AVIUM (Turkey bordatellosis. Turkey coryza)
Vaccine Type: ML bacteria
Information: For turkeys. WD - 21 days. Do not use 10 days before or after another live bacterial or viral vaccine. Vaccinate by the eye drop method at one day of age and again at two weeks of age by the drinking water method. Revaccinate every 4 to 6 weeks as needed according to the exposure conditions.

COCCIDIOSIS (various *Eimeria* species)
Vaccine Type: Live organism. Separate chicken and turkey vaccines; C
Information: Chickens and Turkeys. Add vaccine to feed or water of very young chicks to produce controlled infection which induces an immunity.

ENCEPHALOMYELITIS VIRUS
Vaccine Type: K, ML. MV or C
Information: Chickens and turkeys. K - vaccinate between 16 and 24 weeks of age, but not before 12 weeks. Revaccinate during molting.
ML - vaccinate between 10 and 18 weeks of age by wing web or drinking water method. Do not save eggs until six weeks after vaccination is given to breeders. Do not vaccinate within 4 weeks of initial egg production nor within 21 days of slaughter.

ERYSIPELOTHRIX RHUSIOPATIAE (Erysipelas)
Vaccine Type: K or ML. MV
Information: Vaccines labeled for turkeys. ML is an oral vaccine and is used in 8 weeks or older turkeys. It is boosted in 2 to 3 weeks and then every 3 months. K vaccines are given by body weight or age and are boosted every 3 months. WD - 21 days for slaughter.

ESCHERICHIA COLI (Colibacillosis. Colisepticemia)
Vaccine Type: K. MV
Information: Chickens and turkeys. Begin vaccinating chickens 2 to 3 weeks of age and turkeys at 1 day. A second vaccination is required. Vaccinate breeding hens 4 weeks prior to laying. WD - 6 weeks for slaughter.

FOWL POX VIRUS
Vaccine Type: ML. MV or C
Information: WD - 21 days. Some vaccines for chickens and some for chickens and turkeys. Given by wing web application in one day old chicks or older depending on vaccine. Turkeys are usually vaccinated at 6 weeks of age or older. Some vaccines recommend boosters.

HAEMOPHILUS PARAGALLINARUM
Vaccine Type: K. MV
Information: For chickens. Vaccinate at 3 to 8 weeks of age depending on vaccine used and boost in 3 to 4 weeks. Some vaccines recommend the booster not be given within 4 weeks of laying. WD - 21 to 42 days depending on vaccine.

HERPESVIRUS (Marek's disease)
Vaccine Type: Live virus
Information: For chickens. Vaccinate one day old chicks. WD - 21 days for slaughter. Most vaccines require liquid nitrogen storage.

INFECTIOUS BRONCHITIS VIRUS
Vaccine Type: K, ML. MV or C
Information: Chickens only. The bronchitis virus in the flock or area needs to be identified in order to vaccinate against the right one. Some vaccines require liquid nitrogen storage. K vaccine can be used in 3 weeks or older chicks, although many vaccines recommend the vaccine to be given at 16 to 22 weeks. Also, many vaccines recommend that a ML vaccine be given 3 to 4 weeks prior to the K vaccine. WD - 42 days for slaughter.
ML: Two options. (1) Vaccinate at 1 day old by injection, boost in 2 weeks and again at 16 to 18 weeks for replacement birds. (2) Vaccinate at 4 to 5 weeks of age by drinking water method. Vaccinate broilers twice and layers again at 16 to 20 weeks. Vaccination methods are by water, intranasal or by eye drop. WD - 21 days for slaughter.

INFECTIOUS BURSAL DISEASE VIRUS (Infectious bursal disease. Gumboro disease)
Vaccine Type: K, ML. MV or C
Information: Chickens only.
K: Vaccinate at 16 weeks of age or older. Some vaccines recommend birds should be primed with ML vaccine at least 4

weeks prior to vaccination. Some vaccines recommend a booster at molting. WD - 42 days for slaughter.
ML: Requires liquid nitrogen storage and is given to one day old chicks. WD - 21 days for slaughter.

INFLUENZA TYPE H1 VIRUS (Fowl plague)
Vaccine Type: K. MV
Information: For turkeys. It is best to vaccinate between 20 to 28 weeks of age and boost in 4 to 6 weeks. WD - 42 days.

LARYNGOTRACHEITIS VIRUS (Infectious laryngotracheitis)
Vaccine Type: ML. MV
Information: Chickens only. In an outbreak chicks can be vaccinated at 10 to 14 days of age. WD - 21 days for slaughter. Under normal conditions vaccinate at 4 weeks and boost in 6 to 12 weeks.

MYCOPLASMA GALLISEPTIUSM (PPLO infection. Chronic respiratory disease. Infectious sinusitis)
Vaccine Type: K or ML. MV or C
Information: For chickens or turkeys. WD - 42 days for slaughter. Do not vaccinate birds just prior to or during egg laying. Some vaccines can be given SQ at one week of age or older or IM at 10 weeks of age or older. Some recommend boosters after 4 weeks and then at molting.
ML: Chickens only. Requires liquid nitrogen storage. WD - 21 days for slaughter. Designed for spray application on chicks older than 6 to 9 weeks depending on the vaccine.

NEWCASTLE DISEASE (Avian pneumoencephalitis)
Vaccine Type: K or live virus. MV or C
Information: For chickens and turkeys. Killed vaccine should be used when other infections are present in the flock. Killed vaccines are also used in conjunction with or as boosters to ML vaccines containing the B1 strain of the virus. WD - 42 days for slaughter.
ML - Initial vaccination at one day, two weeks or four weeks of age, depending on vaccine used. Boosters required. Some are for drinking water or spray on administration, some are given by SC injection and others are given intranasally or dropped on the eye. Some vaccines require liquid nitrogen storage. WD - 21 days.

PARAMYXOVIRUS TYPE 3
Vaccine Type: K. MV
Information: Turkeys only. Vaccinate between 20 and 24 weeks of age is recommended although it can be done at any age. Revaccinate 4 to 6 weeks later. WD - 42 days for slaughter.

PASTEURELLA MULTOCIDA (Fowl cholera)
Vaccine Type: K, ML. MV or C
Information: WD - 21 to 42 days depending on vaccine. Chickens and turkeys. Begin vaccinating turkeys at 6 to 10 weeks of age depending on vaccine. Boost at 5 to 12 week intervals depending on vaccine. Some oral vaccines are available for turkeys.

REOVIRUS (Viral arthritis. Tenosynovitis)
Vaccine Type: K or ML. MV or C
Information: K: Chickens only. Same as infectious bursal disease virus.
ML: Some vaccines are for made for drinking water administrations to chicks 2 weeks old or greater. WD - 21 days for slaughter. Some vaccines are used in day old chicks and require liquid nitrogen storage. Some vaccines can be given at 5 days of age with boosters at 5 to 6 weeks and again at 9 to 11 weeks of age. Other vaccines require vaccination once at 3 to 18 weeks of age.

BOVINE VACCINATIONS

Information for bovine vaccines was compounded from Compendium of Veterinary Products, K. Bennett, B.S., 1993, unless indicated by suprascript.

FORMAT AND ABBREVIATIONS

Name of microorganism and/or names of associated diseases:

Vaccine Type:	L	- live vaccine
	K	- killed vaccine
	ML	- modified live vaccine
	SU	- subunit vaccine
	MV	- monovalent (microorganism is the only one in vaccine)
	C	- Compound (multiple microorganisms are in vaccine)
Information:	WD	- withdrawal period

AKABANE[21] (Curly lamb disease, curly calf disease, dummy calf disease)

Vaccine Type: ML & K from Japan. K from Australia.

Information: Vaccines induce immunity in the cow or ewe and circulating antibodies prevent the virus from reaching the fetus.

ANAPLASMOSIS (*Anaplasma marginale*)

Vaccine Type: K. MV

Information: Not recommended for pregnant cows. 60 day WD. Vaccinate cattle twice at not less than 4 weeks apart. Give a booster the following year and then every 2 years. Antibiotics can be administered at the same time.

ANTHRAX (*Bacillus anthracis*, Splenic Fever, Charbon, Milzbrand)

Vaccine Type: ML. MV

Information: Consult a physician upon accidental exposure to vaccine. 60 day WD. All domesticated farm animals are susceptible to infection. In endemic areas vaccinate prior to usual time of outbreaks. Boost in 2-3 weeks and annually.

BRUCELLA ABORTUS (Brucellosis, Bang's Disease, Contagious Abortion)

Vaccine Type: Live - Strain 19 or RB-51. MV

Information: Human exposure to vaccine can cause undulant fever - any exposure should result in immediate care by a physician. Burn unused and empty containers. Vaccinating heifers at 4 to 8 months of age is best, but follow the guidelines set by the local animal health authorities. Do not vaccinate bulls. 21 day WD for strain 19. 12 week WD for RB-51.

BVD (Bovine Viral Diarrhea Virus, Mucosal Disease)
Vaccine Type: ML, K. MV or C
Information: ML - not intended for use in pregnant cows or calves less than 2 months of age.

CAMPYLOBACTER FETUS (Vibriosis, infertility, abortion)
Vaccine Type: K. MV or C
Information: Vaccinate cows 14-28 days prior to breeding.

CLOSTRIDIUM CHAUVOEI (Blackleg)
CLOSTRIDIUM HEMOLYTICUM (Red water)
CLOSTRIDIUM NOVYI (Blacks disease, Infectious necrotic hepatitis)
CLOSTRIDIUM PERFRINGENS TYPES C AND D(Enterotoxemia, Overeating disease)
CLOSTRIDIUM SEPTICUM (Malignant edema)
CLOSTRIDIUM SORDELII
CLOSTRIDIUM TETANI (Lockjaw)
Vaccine Type: K, toxoids, antitoxin to tetanus and Cl. perfringens type C and D. MV or C
Information: Some of the clostridial diseases infect the very young, so vaccinating the cow in the last trimester is recommended. Calves should begin vaccinations as early as 2 months of age. Annual boosters recommended. Antitoxin for tetanus should be given at time of castration and/or dehorn.

CORONAVIRUS (Calfhood diarrhea)
Vaccine Type: K, ML, antiserum. C
Information: ML is given to day old calves or cows in late pregnancy with 2 doses 3-6 weeks apart. Antiserum is given to newborn calves less than 12 hours old. K is given to cows prior to calving in 2 doses with last given within 40 days of calving.

CORYNEBACTERIUM PYOGENES (Calf pneumonia)
Vaccine Type: Antiserum. C
Information: Antiserum is to prevent or treat pneumonia in calves or cattle.

E. COLI (*Escherichia coli,* Enteric colibacillosis)
Vaccine Type: K, Antiserum. MV or C
Information: Antiserum is given to newborn calves in the first 12 hours for prevention or as needed for treatment. K vaccine is given to cows in 2 doses prior to calving.

FOOT AND MOUTH DISEASE[21]
Vaccine Type: K: There are two types, (1) aluminum hydroxide - saponin adjuvanted and (2) oil adjuvanted.
Information: The oil adjuvanted vaccine produces a longer lasting immunity.

FUSOBACTERIUM NECROPHORUM (Foot rot)
Vaccine Type: K. MV
Information: 2 doses required 3-4 weeks apart. Boosters required annually or in endemic conditions where disease is likely to break.

HEMOPHILUS SOMNUS (part of bovine respiratory disease complex, abortion, weak calf syndrome, thromboembolic meningo-encephalitis, TEME)
Vaccine Type: K. MV or C
Information: Begin vaccinating calves at 3 months. Certain compound vaccines can be used in pregnant cows. Boost in 2-4 weeks and annually. Calves vaccinated under 6 months should be boosted at 6 months or at weaning.

IBR (Bovine herpesvirus 1, respiratory disease, abortions, genital infection, systemic disease, encephalitis, conjunctivitis)
Vaccine Type: ML or K. MV or C
Information: ML is not intended for pregnant cows, nursing calves or calves less than 2 months of age. ML is one dose repeated at 6 months of age or at weaning in young calves. For K vaccine follow directions under Haemophilus.

LEPTOSPIROSIS (*L. hardjo, L. pomona, L. grippotyphosa, L. canicola, L. icterohaemorrhagiae.* Redwater of calves, abortion, still birth, lowered milk production)
Vaccine Type: K. MV - pomona only, C - all five types
Information: Single dose initially with annual boosters.

MORAXELLA BOVIS (Pinkeye, Infectious Bovine Keratoconjunctivitis, IBK)
Vaccine Type: K. MV or C
Information: Vaccinate annually prior to season.

PAPILLOMA VIRUS (Warts)
Vaccine Type: K. MV
Information: Used for treating warts.

PASTEURELLA (*P. multocida, P. haemolytica.* Shipping fever, transit fever, part of bovine respiratory disease complex, haemorrhagic septicemia)
Vaccine Type: K, Antiserum, ML. MV or C
Information: ML - Vaccinate calves 3 months of age or older. Boost annually. Not for use in pregnant cows or calves less than 3 months old.
K - Same instructions as hemophilus somnus. Antiserum is used for treating sick animals.

PI3 (Parainfluenza 3 virus, part of bovine respiratory disease complex, bovine viral pneumonia)
Vaccine Type: ML, K. C
Information: Same as IBR.

RABIES
Vaccine Type: K
Information: Vaccinate annually those 3 months of age and older.

RESPIRATORY SYNCYTIAL VIRUS (Part of bovine respiratory disease complex)
Vaccine Type: K, ML. MV or C
Information: Same instructions as hemophilus somnus. ML - not intended for use in pregnant cows.

RIFT VALLEY FEVER[21] (Infectious enzootic hepatitis of sheep and cattle)
Information: K vaccine requires 2 inoculations for protection and annual boosters.
ML (mutagen - attenuated vero cell - propagated vaccine) has been developed for use in people and tested in sheep and cattle. This vaccine causes no adverse effects in lambs or calves or pregnant sheep or cattle. One inoculation provides rapid immunity.

RINDERPEST[21] (Cattle plague, peste bovina)
Vaccine Type: There are two ML vaccines. The goat adapted vaccine (GRV) is not safe for animals with low innate resistance or harboring latent infections. GRV is also lethal for sheep and goats. The cell culture adapted vaccine (TCRV) is safe and can be used in all species in which it has been tested.
Information: Calves with little or no maternally derived antibody and adult cattle obtain a solid, long-term immunity. Calves between 4 and 6 months of age should be vaccinated annually for 3 consecutive years to ensure a protective level of immunity.

ROTAVIRUS (Calfhood Diarrhea)
Vaccine Type: K, ML. Antiserum. C
Information: Same as coronavirus.

SALMONELLA TYPHIMURIUM
Vaccine Type: K, Antiserum, K/toxoid combo. MV, C
Information: Antiserum used in treatment of sick animals. K - initial vaccination requires 2 doses 2-4 weeks apart. Vaccinate pregnant cows 4-6 weeks before calving. Annual boosters needed.

STAPHYLOCOCCUS AUREAS (Staphylococcal mastitis)
Vaccine Type: K. MV or C
Information: Initial vaccination requires 2 doses at 14 day intervals. Boost every 6 months to one year. It is best to time 2 boosters at 3-6 weeks before calving.

TRICHOMONA FOETUS (infertility, early fetal death)
Vaccine Type: K Protozoa. MV or C
Information: Initial vaccination requires 2 doses at 2-4 week intervals with the second given at 4 weeks prior to breeding season. Annual booster recommended.

CANINE VACCINES

Information for canine vaccines was taken from Infectious Diseases of the Dog and Cat, 1990, W.B. Saunders Co., Craig E. Greene; with additional information from the Compendium of Veterinary Products, K. Bennett, B.S., 1993.

FORMAT AND ABBREVIATIONS

Name of microorganism and/or names of associated diseases:

Vaccine Type: L - live vaccine
K - killed vaccine
ML - modified live vaccine
SU - subunit vaccine
MV- monovalent (microorganism is the only one in vaccine)
C - Compound (multiple microorganisms are in vaccine)

Information: WD - withdrawal period

ADENOVIRUS (Infectious canine hepatitis = ICH)

Vaccine Type: K, ML. C

Information: Adenovirus-1 is the etiologic cause of ICH. In a small number of dogs ML Adenovirus-1 can cause persistent kidney infection or eye problems including uveitis or corneal opacity (blue eye). Adenovirus-2 can cause respiratory infection. ML Adenovirus-2 cross protects against ICH.

Same administration routine as distemper.

BORDATELLA BRONCHISEPTICA (Part of Infectious tracheobronchitis complex)

Vaccine Type: K, ML. MV, C

Information: Same as parainfluenza virus.

BORRELIA BERGDORFERI (Lyme disease)

Vaccine Type: K. MV, C

Information: Give two doses three weeks apart to dogs older than 12 weeks. Give IM.

CORONAVIRUS (Coronaviral enteritis)

Vaccine Type: K. MV, C

Information: Vaccinate beginning at 6 weeks of age, giving boosters every 2-3 weeks with last vaccine given at 12 weeks of age or later. Boost annually or in the midst of an outbreak.

DISTEMPTER VIRUS
Vaccine Type: ML canine distemper virus. MV, C
Information: Vaccinate every 3-4 weeks beginning at 6-8 weeks of age (2-3 weeks of age if pups were colostrum deprived). Final vaccination should be at 12 weeks or later. Boost annually.

LEPTOSPIROSIS (*Leptospira canicola* and *L. icterohaemorrhagiae*).
Vaccine Type: K. C
Information: Vaccinate beginning at 9 weeks of age and boost 3 times at 2-3 week intervals. Duration of immunity is 6-12 months. Vaccinating prior to 9 weeks is not recommended because of the allergic nature of the vaccine. The allergic reaction is usually seen within minutes to hours after the booster is given. Local or systemic symptoms are seen - skin wheals, vomiting, facial swelling, diarrhea, difficulty breathing, collapse or even death. Treat with epinephrine and corticosteroids.

MEASLES VIRUS
Vaccine Type: ML. C
Information: Designed to protect young puppies against distemper virus infection. Usually used only for the first vaccination. Do not give to adult females used for breeding.

PARAINFLUENZA VIRUS (Part of Infectious tracheobronchitis complex)
Vaccine Type: ML. C
Information: Same vaccination regimen as distemper. Intranasal vaccines are available and possibly give quicker immunity and a better immunity in the nasal passages.

PARVOVIRUS (Parvoviral Enteritis)
Vaccine Type: K, ML. MV, C
Information: ML feline origin parvoviral vaccines are less effective than those of ML canine origin. Killed vaccines should be used in pups less than 5 weeks old and in pregnant bitches (2 doses in 1st trimester). Vaccines should be given every 3-4 weeks with last vaccine given at 18 weeks of age or older.

RABIES VIRUS (Hydrophobia)
Vaccine Type: K. MV
Information: Vaccinate at 3 months of age and 1 year later. Boost every 1-3 years depending on vaccine used and recommendations of local health authorities. Give IM in one spot in the thigh unless otherwise indicated on the label.

CAPRINE VACCINES

Unless indicated by suprascript, information on caprine vaccines was taken from the Council Report, "Vaccination Guidelines for Small Ruminants", JAVMA, vol. 205, no. 11, December 1, 1994.

FORMAT AND ABBREVIATIONS

Name of microorganism and/or names of associated diseases:

Vaccine Type:	L	- live vaccine
	K	- killed vaccine
	ML	- modified live vaccine
	SU	- subunit vaccine
	MV	- monovalent (microorganism is the only one in vaccine)
	C	- Compound (multiple microorganisms are in vaccine)
Information:	WD	- withdrawal period

BACTEROIDES NODUSUS - Not routinely used in goats.

BLUE TONGUE - Not routinely used in goats.

CHLAMYDIA PSITTACI - Used in goats for unlicensed purposes. For information see ovine vaccines.

CLOSTRIDIA:

CL. CHAUVOEI (Big head, Blackleg)

CL. HEMOLYTICUM (Redwater)

CL. PERFRINGENS TYPES C AND D (Enterotoxemia, Struck, Overeating disease, Pulpy kidney disease)

CL. SEPTICUM (Braxy, Malignant edema)

CL. TETANI (Lockjaw)

Products are available for these clostridia which are licensed for goats. For information see ovine vaccines.

CONTAGIOUS ECTHYMA - Products available for goats. For information see ovine vaccines.

CORYNEBACTEERIUM PSEUDOTUBERCULOSIS - Used in goats for unlicensed purposes. See ovine vaccines for information.

GOAT AND SHEEP POX - See information under sheep pox under ovine vaccines.

PESTE DES PETITS RUMINANTS[21] (Pest of small ruminants, pseudorinderpest of small ruminants)

Information: Bovine rinderpest vaccine has been used successfully to impart immunity. Testing is being done on an ML vaccine specifically for peste des petits ruminants.

RABIES - Used in goats for unlicensed purposes.

RINDERPEST[21] - Vaccination with the cattle rinderpest vaccine has been reported. See information under cattle vaccines.

TETANUS ANTITOXIN (Lockjaw)

Vaccine Type: Antiserum

Information: (1) For treatment of tetanus give 100-1000 U/kg IV, IM or SC as a one time treatment. 20,000 U is maximum dose. IV administration given slowly over 5-10 minutes is best, although allergic reactions are possible. Have corticosteroids and antihistamines ready or pretreat with them. Giving 1000 U at and around the wound site may prove helpful. (2) For prevention give 500 U SQ.

EQUINE VACCINES

Information for equine vaccines was compounded from Compendium of Veterinary Products, K. Bennett, B.S., 1993, unless indicated by suprascript.

FORMAT AND ABBREVIATIONS

Name of microorganism and/or names of associated diseases:

Vaccine Type: L - live vaccine
K - killed vaccine
ML - modified live vaccine
SU - subunit vaccine
MV - monovalent (microorganism is the only one in vaccine)
C - Compound (multiple microorganisms are in vaccine)

Information: WD - withdrawal period

AFRICAN HORSE SICKNESS[21]

Information: ML vaccine (quadrivalent) given as two doses three weeks apart.

ANTHRAX - See information under cattle vaccines.

E. COLI (*Escherichia coli*)

Vaccine Type: Antiserum

Information: Administer to foals within 12 hours of birth.

ENCEPHALOMYELITIS (Equine encephalitis, Brain fever, Sleeping sickness. Eastern, Western and Venezuelan encephalomyelitis viruses)

Vaccine Type: K. C

Information: Initial vaccination requires 2 doses 3-4 weeks apart. Annual boosters required. In endemic areas foals are to be vaccinated at 3, 4 and 6 months of age.

INFLUENZA (Equine influenza viruses subtypes A1 and A2)

Vaccine Type: K, MV. C

Information: Begin vaccinating at 3 months of age. Initial series requires 2 doses 3-4 weeks apart. Boost annually and whenever epidemic conditions exist or exposure is likely up to every 3 months.

RHINOPNEUMONITIS (Equine herpesvirus 1 subtypes 1 and 2, Equine respiratory disease, Equine abortion virus)
Vaccine Type: K, ML. MV, C
Information: K vaccine is used to prevent abortions. It is given at 5, 7 and 9 months of the pregnancy. K vaccine can be used in young horses to prevent respiratory infection by vaccinating with 2 doses initially at 3-4 week intervals, followed by boosters after 6 months and then annually. Also boost whenever epidemic conditions exist or exposure is likely.
ML is used to prevent respiratory infection. Vaccinate horses older than 3 months with 2 initial doses at 4-8 week intervals. Boost every 3 months.
Immunity from K or ML is short lived (2-4 months).

SALMONELLA TYPHIMURIUM
Vaccine Type: Antiserum, K. MV
Information: Antiserum is used to prevent or treat salmonella endotoxemia. K vaccine is given initially in 2 doses at 2-3 week intervals. Annual booster recommended.

STREPTOCOCCUS EQUI (Strangles, Distemper, Barn fever)
Vaccine Type: K. MV
Information: Vaccinate horses 3 months of age or older with 3 doses at 2-4 week intervals. Annual booster recommended.

TETANUS (*Clostridium tetani*, Lockjaw)
Vaccine Type: Toxoid, Antitoxin
Information: Toxoid is used to stimulate the immune system. Antitoxin provides immediate protection in face of injury and is also used in massive doses in treatment of tetanus. Toxoid is given initially in 2 doses at a 3-4 week interval to foals over 3 months of age. Boost annually!

VIRAL ARTERITIS (Equine typhoid, abortion, respiratory disease)
Vaccine Type: ML. MV
Information: Vaccinate foals older than 6 weeks. Vaccinate stallions and brood mares at least 3 weeks prior to breeding. One dose required. Not recommended for use in pregnant mares unless threatened by natural exposure.

FELINE VACCINES

Information for feline vaccines was taken from Infectious Diseases of the Dog and Cat, 1990, W.B. Saunders Co., Craig E. Greene; with additional information from the Compendium of Veterinary Products, K. Bennett, B.S., 1993.

FORMAT AND ABBREVIATIONS

Name of microorganism and/or names of associated diseases:

Vaccine Type:	L	- live vaccine
	K	- killed vaccine
	ML	- modified live vaccine
	SU	- subunit vaccine
	MV	- monovalent (microorganism is the only one in vaccine)
	C	- Compound (multiple microorganisms are in vaccine)
Information:	WD	- withdrawal period

CALICIVIRUS AND RHINOTRACHEITIS VIRUS (Feline respiratory disease)

Vaccine Type: ML and K for parenteral use and ML for intranasal (IN) use. C

Information: 2 parenteral doses needed 3-4 weeks apart beginning at 8 weeks of age with the last given at 12 weeks or greater. IN vaccine may provide protection in 48 hours. IN vaccines may induce a mild contagious respiratory illness. Boost annually or in midst of outbreak. Immunity probably is incomplete and of variable length.

CHLAMYDIA PSITTACI (Pneumonitis)

Vaccine Type: K, ML. MV, C

Information: Vaccine offers incomplete immunity. Vaccinate every 3-4 weeks beginning at 8 weeks with the last given at 12 weeks of age or greater. For cats older than 12 weeks one vaccination should be sufficient. Annual boosters needed.

FIP (Feline infectious peritonitis virus)

Vaccine Type: ML. MV

Information: Intranasal administration. Begin vaccinating at 16 weeks of age, boost in 3 to 4 weeks. Boost annually.

LEUKEMIA (Feline viral leukemia)
Vaccine Type: K, SU. MV, C
Information: Pre-vaccination testing is recommended. Occult infections exist which are undetectable by current tests. Vaccination is not 100% protective. Begin vaccinating at 8 to 10 weeks of age and boost in 2-4 weeks depending on product.

PANLEUKOPENIA VIRUS (Distemper)
Vaccine Type: K, ML. MV, C
Information: At least 2-ML or 3-K vaccines should be given at 3-4 week intervals beginning at 8 weeks of age with last given at 12 weeks or more. Annual boosters recommended.

RABIES - See canine information.

LLAMA VACCINES

Information on llama vaccines was taken from the Council Report, "Vaccination Guidelines for Small Ruminants", JAVMA, vol. 205, no. 11, December 1, 1994.

FORMAT AND ABBREVIATIONS

Name of microorganism and/or names of associated diseases:

Vaccine Type:	L	- live vaccine
	K	- killed vaccine
	ML	- modified live vaccine
	SU	- subunit vaccine
	MV	- monovalent (microorganism is the only one in vaccine)
	C	- Compound (multiple microorganisms are in vaccine)
Information:	WD	- withdrawal period

There are no licensed products for llamas in the United States. Use of vaccines should be under the direction of a licensed veterinarian.

BVD (Bovine viral diarrhea)

Information: Use a killed vaccine annually.

CHLAMYDIA (Ovine enzootic abortion)

Information: Use a killed vaccine annually prior to breeding. Systemic and local reactions may occur. Killed product is combined with ***Campylobacter*** or with ***Campylobacter*** and ***E. coli***.

CLOSTRIDIUM PERFRINGENS TYPES C AND D*

Vaccine Type: K given IM or SC.

Information: Pregnant females - 4 weeks before birthing. Give to crias at 2-3 months and again at 4-6 months, followed by annual boosters. Give to adults annually. Antitoxins are given to cria if dam is not vaccinated.

CL. TETANI*

Vaccine Type: Toxoid given IM or SC.

Information: Can be given at 1 week of age, followed by 2 doses 3-4 weeks apart with annual boosters. Pregnant females - 4 weeks prior to birthing.

CL. CHAUVOEI AND CL. SEPTICUM* - Same as for sheep.

CL. NOVYI, CL. HEMOLYTICUM AND CL. SORDELLI* - Same as for sheep.
Information: Questions exist as to whether these are useful in llamas. They may be indicated if liver flukes are a problem.

*There are reports of abortions in llamas following administration of "7/8/9 Way" combinations of clostridial vaccines. Therefore, administration of these products to pregnant animals may not be indicated.

CORONAVIRUS
Vaccine Type: Use the K bovine vaccine.

ECTHYMA
Vaccine Type: L virus.
Information: Use only in diseased herd or in an outbreak.

E. COLI (diarrhea in cria)
Vaccine Type: K (see ***Chlamydia***)
Information: Vaccine given to dams 4 weeks prior to birthing.

EQUINE HERPES VIRUS-1
Vaccine Type: K vaccine given SC
Information: Vaccinate every 12 weeks. May be indicated if llamas are kept near horses or related species.

IBR (Infectious bovine rhinotracheitis)
Information: Use K vaccine IM annually.

LEPTOSPIROSIS INTERROGANS (L. icterohaemorrhagiae, L. canicola, L. grippotyphosa, L. hardjo, L. pomona)
Information: Use where disease is endemic. Vaccinate as often as 3-4 times per year.

RABIES
Vaccine Type: K vaccine (hamster embryo "lines")
Information: Vaccinate annually as early as 3 months of age. Vaccinated animals should be considered non-vaccinated if exposed.

ROTAVIRUS
Vaccine Type: Use the K bovine vaccine.

OVINE VACCINES

Unless indicated by suprascript, information on ovine vaccines was taken from the Council Report, "Vaccination Guidelines for Small Ruminants", JAVMA, vol. 205, no. 11, December 1, 1994 and Compendium of Veterinary Products, K. Bennett, B. S., 1993.

FORMAT AND ABBREVIATIONS

Name of microorganism and/or names of associated diseases:

Vaccine Type:	L	- live vaccine
	K	- killed vaccine
	ML	- modified live vaccine
	SU	- subunit vaccine
	MV	- monovalent (microorganism is the only one in vaccine)
	C	- Compound (multiple microorganisms are in vaccine)
Information:	WD	- withdrawal period

AKABANE[21] - See information under cattle vaccines.

ANTHRAX - See information under cattle vaccines. Give SQ.

BACTEROIDES NODOSUS (Footrot)
Vaccine Type: K. MV
Information: Give SC. Initial vaccination requires 2 doses with second given between 6 weeks and 6 months after the first. Boost every 4-6 months in cases of severe challenge. Twice yearly boosters are recommended. Local vaccine reactions are common.

BLUETONGUE (Sore muzzle)
Vaccine Type: ML (type 10 virus). MV
Information: Give SC. Vaccinate prior to biting fly season. Do not vaccinate pregnant animals. Vaccinate 3 weeks prior to breeding or after birthing. Young animals should be vaccinated at 3 months of age.

BRUCELLA OVIS (Ram epididymitis)
Vaccine Type: K. MV
Information: Vaccinate only rams. Use 2 initial doses 4 weeks apart. Questionable efficacy.

CAMPYLOBACTER FETUS, AND C. JEJUNI (Vibriosis, abortion)
Vaccine Type: K. MV, C
Information: Some vaccines require 60 day WD. Two doses are given initially, both prior to breeding. Annual booster recommended. Make sure the product is labeled for sheep.

CHLAMYDIA PSITTACI (Ovine enzootic abortion)
Vaccine Type: K. C
Information: Same as for campylobacter. Local and systemic reactions occur.

CLOSTRIDIA:
CL. CHAUVOEI (Big head, Blackleg)
CL. HEMOLYTICUM (Redwater)
CL. NOVYI (Big head, Black's disease, Infectious necrotic hepatitis)
CL. PERFRINGENS TYPES C AND D (Enterotoxemia, Struck, Overeating disease, Pulpy kidney disease)
CL. SEPTICUM (Braxy, Malignant edema)
CL. SORDELLI (Big head)
CL. TETANI (Lockjaw)
Vaccine Type: K, toxoids, antitoxin to tetanus and *Cl. perfringens* type C and D. C
Information: SQ administration of vaccines is preferable over IM. Antitoxin to Cl. perfringens type C and D is used in outbreaks. K vaccine of Cl. perfringens types C and D can be given to one week old lambs from unvaccinated ewes. Antitoxin for tetanus should be given at time of castration, dehorn and tail dock. Some clostridial diseases infect the very young, therefore, vaccinating the ewe in late pregnancy is recommended. In general, lambs can be vaccinated at 2 months of age. Annual boosters recommended.

CORYNEBACTERIUM PSEUDOTUBERCULOSIS
Vaccine Type: K with toxoid. MV, C
Information: Give SQ. Two doses initial vaccination with second dose 4 weeks after first. Revaccinate annually. Local and systemic reactions occur. Do not use in known infected animals.

E. COLI

Vaccine Type: Antiserum, K. MV or C

Information: K - Same instructions as for campylobacter.
Antiserum - for prevention and treatment of colibacillosis in newborn lambs - give in first 12 hours of life.

ECTHYMA (Sore mouth)

Vaccine Type: L. MV

Information: Give SQ. Vaccinate each new lamb crop and new additions to flock. The vaccine is brushed onto scarified skin. Vaccine may cause the disease "orf" in humans. Vaccine must be handled and disposed of properly.

PASTEURELLA HAEMOLYTICA, P. MULTOCIDA (Part of Shipping fever complex)

Vaccine Type: K, Antiserum. C

Information: Antiserum is used in treatment of sick animals.
K - Vaccinate twice at 2-4 week intervals. Animals vaccinated initially at less than 3 months of age should be boosted at 4-6 months of age.

RABIES (Hydrophobia)

Vaccine Type: K, MV

Information: Give IM. Vaccinate annually those 3 months of age and older.

RINDERPEST[21] - Vaccination with the cattle rinderpest vaccine has been reported. See information under cattle vaccines.

SALMONELLA TYPHIMURIUM

Vaccine Type: Antiserum

Information: Used in treatment of sick animals.

SHEEP AND GOAT POX[21]

Information: K vaccines do not provide a long lasting immunity. ML vaccines such as the Romanian strain or the Kenya O 180 strain have been used effectively.

TETANUS - See Clostridia.

PORCINE VACCINES

Information for porcine vaccines was compounded from Compendium of Veterinary Products, K. Bennett, B. S., 1993, unless indicated by suprascript.

FORMAT AND ABBREVIATIONS

Name of microorganism and/or names of associated diseases:

Vaccine Type:	L	- live vaccine
	K	- killed vaccine
	ML	- modified live vaccine
	SU	- subunit vaccine
	MV	- monovalent (microorganism is the only one in vaccine)
	C	- Compound (multiple microorganisms are in vaccine)
Information:	WD	- withdrawal period

ANTHRAX - See information under cattle vaccines.

BORDATELLA BRONCHISEPTICA (Atrophic rhinitis)

Vaccine Type: K, ML. MV or C

Information: All ages can be vaccinated. Intranasal vaccines are given to piglets. Sows are given 2 doses prior to farrowing. Boost annually prior to farrowing.

CLOSTRIDIA

***CL. PERFRINGENS* TYPE C** (Piglet Enterotoxemia)

***CL. NOVYI* TOXOID** (Infectious Necrotic Hepatitis)

CL. SEPTICUM (Malignant Edema)

CL. TETANI (Lockjaw)

Vaccine Type: K, Toxoids, Antiserum for Tetanus. MV or C

Information: Clostridial diseases are less common in pigs compared to other species. Vaccinate sows in last trimester to help prevent piglet enterotoxemia. Vaccinations for other clostridial diseases are usually done in the midst of problems or in the case of tetanus antitoxin at the time of castration or injury.

E. COLI (Escherichia coli, Colibacillosis)
Vaccine Type: K, Antiserum. MV or C
Information: Vaccinate sows twice prior to farrowing. Boost annually prior to farrowing. Antiserum is given to piglets less than 12 hours old.

ENCEPHALOMYOCARDITIS VIRUS
Vaccine Type: K. MV
Information: Vaccinates sows twice prior to farrowing. Vaccinate boars twice 2-3 weeks apart and then semi-annually. 60 day WD before slaughter.

ERISIPELOTHRIX RHUSIOPATHIAE (Erysipelas)
Vaccine Type: K, ML, Antiserum. MV or C
Information: Antiserum is given to healthy pigs in the midst of an outbreak or to sick pigs as a part of the treatment. Some ML vaccines can also be given orally to piglets. K products should be given twice at 2-3 week intervals.

HAEMOPHILUS PLEUROPNEUMONIAE (Actinobacillus)
Vaccine Type: K
Information: Vaccinate pigs twice 2-4 weeks apart. Vaccinate sows prior to farrowing. Annual boosters recommended.

HOG CHOLERA[21]
Information: Good ML vaccines are available and can be used in pregnant sows and piglets over 2 weeks old.

LEPTOSPIROSIS (*L. canicola, L. grippotyphosa, L. hardjo, L. icterohaemorrhagiae, L. pomona*)
Vaccine Type: K. MV (pomona only) or C
Information: Vaccinate sows and gilts twice prior to breeding, then prior to subsequent breedings. Boars are vaccinated at greater than 8 months with semi-annual boosters.

MYCOPLASMA HYOPNEUMONIAE
Vaccine Type: K. MV or C
Information: Vaccinate at one week or older. Boost in 2-4 weeks. Sows and gilts are best vaccinated or boosted prior to farrowing. Annual or semi-annual re-vaccination is required.

PARVOVIRUS (SMEDI)
Vaccine Type: K. MV or C
Information: Vaccinate sows and gilts 14-60 days prior to breeding with gilts best protected when vaccinated 14 days prior to breeding. Some vaccines require booster in 14-28 days. Re-vaccinate prior to subsequent breedings.

PASTEURELLA MULTOCIDA (Atrophic rhinitis)
Vaccine Type: K. MV or C
Information: Same as those for Haemophilus.

PSEUDORABIES (Herpesvirus, Aujesky's Disease, Mad Itch)
Vaccine Type: ML or K
Information: Young pigs can be vaccinated and should be boosted at 10-12 weeks of age. Sows and boars require an initial vaccination with semi-annual to annual boosters prior to farrowing.

ROTAVIRUS
Vaccine Type: K or ML. MV or C
Information: WD for K products is 60 days.
IM Method: Vaccinate sows and gilts twice prior to farrowing. 1-2 boosters required for each subsequent farrowing. Some vaccines can be given orally to unexposed swine. Some vaccines can be given to piglets.

SALMONELLA CHOLERASUIS and ***SALMONELLA TYPHIMURIUM***
Vaccine Type: K. MV
Information: Give 2 doses 2-4 weeks apart to pregnant sows and gilts prior to farrowing. To piglets give 2 doses 2-4 weeks apart with the first doses given at weaning. Some vaccines require 60 day WD.

SERVULINA (Treponema) ***HYODYSENTERIAE*** (Swine Dysentery)
Vaccine Type: K. MV
Information: Vaccinate piglets twice 3 weeks apart beginning at 8 weeks of age. Boosters are recommended in an outbreak.

STREPTOCOCCUS SUIS
Vaccine Type: K, Antiserum. MV or C
Information: Same as haemophilus except boost every 6 months. Some vaccines require 60 day WD. Antiserum is used for prevention and treatment during an outbreak.

TETANUS - See clostridia.

TGE VIRUS (Transmissible gastroenteritis)
Vaccine Type: K or ML. MV or C
Information: Vaccinate sows and gilts twice before farrowing. Some vaccines can be given to baby piglets. Some vaccines can be given orally. Some vaccines require 60 day WD.

SECTION 9

CONTROL OF ECTOPARASITES

CONTROL OF ECTOPARASITES

INTRODUCTION

Ectoparasites are those pests that spend all or part of their life cycle living on an animal, whether that be bird, mammal or fish. These parasites cause direct loss to producers by damaging hides and muscle tissue, causing anemia due to blood loss, spreading diseases and annoying the host animals which can lead to decreased production.

To minimize damages caused by these pests, it is important to identify the specific parasite and choose the most effective treatment. This treatment, called an ectoparasiticide or insecticide, may come in various forms. Some are applied directly on the animal and others are used in the animal's environment to control the population of the parasite (refer to Methods of Application).

To control ectoparasites it is important to use proper animal husbandry practices, such as spreading manure and soiled bedding lightly on fields so fly eggs and larvae will dry and die. Remove spilled feed and water puddles from animal pens, and watch animals for signs of parasite infestation.

SAFETY RESTRICTIONS

Because insecticides are toxins, they must be used with caution. They can be harmful, and even deadly, to humans and animals, as well as to the parasites themselves. When handling, mixing, applying or disposing of these toxins, always read and follow label instructions carefully. Be very careful not to contaminate the environment, especially the food or water supply in the area by thoughtless disposal of containers or drainage of excess dip from animals. If you have doubts about disposal, store used containers in a safe area until a public health care professional can advise you.

METHODS OF APPLICATION[5, 23]

There are various methods of application depending on the facilities, equipment available and the chemical to be applied.

A. <u>Dipping</u> - A large vat or tank (10,000 liters or 2,500 gallons for cattle) is filled with the chemical solution and each animal is immersed one at a time. For smaller livestock the vat may be smaller and sometimes a metal cage holding the animal may be lowered into the solution. In all cases, the dipped animal should have an area to stand where runoff drains back into the vat.

ADVANTAGES:

Treatment is complete and thorough.

DISADVANTAGES:

1. Only a few insecticides are approved for use in vats.
2. Vats are usually permanent, immovable structures, such as concrete tanks, so animals must be brought to the vat.
3. The initial cost for filling the vat is high.
4. The insecticide must be maintained at the correct dilution by adding more over time.
5. Once the vat contents are contaminated and the insecticide too weak to be effective, the solution must be disposed of properly, as should all chemicals.

B. Spraying - Pump-up or motorized sprayers are used very commonly, especially when treating animals in remote areas or in small numbers.

ADVANTAGES:

1. Portable equipment.
2. No left over chemical to dispose of since you can mix the exact amount needed.

DISADVANTAGES:

1. The equipment and applicator must be sufficient to apply the solution in the proper quantity and at correct pressure (250-300 psi or pounds per square inch).
2. Diluted pesticide may become inactive or hazardous to the animal if allowed to sit for a prolonged time.
3. A good source of water is required since it may require four liters (or one gallon) of spray for each animal.

C. Hand-Application - Small numbers of animals or individual animals may be treated by hand, especially for protecting wounds or preventing fly-strike. Dusts, sprays, ointments, pour-ons and spot-ons may be applied by hand. Pour-on products are poured down the back from shoulders to hips on cattle. Spot-ons are applied to a small area on the back of the animal and are used on cattle, goats, sheep and hogs.

D. Ear Tags and Fly Repellent Strips - Plastic tags and strips infused with insecticide, which is released slowly to provide long-term protection from flies and ticks, may be attached directly to the animal.

ADVANTAGES:

1. Very effective for ear ticks.
2. Can be applied to halter and tail of horses.

DISADVANTAGES:

In some areas, horn flies are resistant to the pyrethroids commonly used in these products.

E. Injections - Subcutaneous injection of appropriate chemicals in the neck region provides systemic action against grubs, mites, sucking lice, as well as intestinal nematodes.

F. Self-Treatment Devices - Back rubbers, dust bags and feed-through insect growth regulators may effectively control some parasites. The back rubber or dust bag is made by wrapping cloth around a cable or rope hung between posts or in a gateway. The cloth is saturated with oil and insecticide solution or filled with insecticide powder. Each time the animal passes under or rubs against these devices, they apply insecticide to their back or face and neck.

These are especially helpful when placed in pathways the animal must frequent, such as to a water, feed or mineral source, thus forcing the animal to apply insecticide several times daily. The dust bags must be kept under a shelter to protect them from the rain. These devices are illustrated in section 6.

Feed additives that contain insect growth regulators are passed in the livestock feces and prevent the fly eggs, which are laid in the feces, from developing into adult flies. However, these products do not kill adult flies which may come from other untreated animals.

CLASSES OF ECTOPARASITICIDES

All chemicals in the same class work in similar ways to kill or inactivate the parasite. Each chemical may be available in various forms and concentrations such as emulsifiable concentrate, wettable powder, pour-on, ear tag, dust, spray foam, injectable and emulsifiable liquid concentrate. Following are some of the major classes of insecticides available today. Be sure to read labels carefully regarding the parasites controlled, the dilution and application instructions and disposal recommendations.

A. Cholinesterase Inhibitors-[5] Also known as acetylcholinesterase inhibitors, these chemicals interfere with normal nerve transmission in the insect so it becomes paralyzed and dies. At high doses it can cause the same action in the livestock as well, so do not use it in combination with other insecticides, or drugs of the same class, or on animals less than 3 months old, or on sick animals. These chemicals are potent and work rapidly. There are two major subgroups of cholinesterase inhibitors: organophosphates and carbamates. Some common organophosphates are: chlorpyriphos, coumaphos, diazinon, dichlorvos, famphur, fenthion, malathion, trichlorfon. Commonly used carbamates are: carbaryl, methomyl and propoxur.

B. **Chlorinated Hydrocarbons**-[24] These chemicals are nervous system stimulants or depressants. Their use has been greatly reduced since the 1970's due to problems with long-term tissue and environmental residue. Do not treat animals that are sick, stressed or under 3 months old. The only chemicals in this class approved for use in livestock now are lindane, methoxychlor and toxaphene. Some of the older compounds which are especially persistent in the environment and animal tissues include DDT, aldrin, heptachlor and chlordane.

C. **Pyrethrins and Synthetic Pyrethroids**-[5, 24] The natural pyrethrins (pyrethrum) are derived from chrysanthemum flowers. The synthetic forms of pyrethrins are called pyrethroids. This class of insecticide works by paralyzing the insect long enough that it dies. The pyrethrins are unstable in air and light and are generally non-toxic to anything other than insects. The new synthetic pyrethroids, however, are more stable and thus more potent to insects and fish. They are still relatively non-toxic to mammals and birds. Some of the most common pyrethroids include: allethrin, fenvalerate, fluvalinate, permethrin and tetramethrin.

D. **Insect Growth Regulators**-[5] These chemicals are not adulticides but they break the life cycle by preventing larvae from developing into adult forms. They are used for fly control in livestock and for flea control in dogs and cats. Methoprene, phenoxycarb and pyriproxyfen are new compounds in the class of insect growth regulators.

E. **Formamidines**-[5] This class of chemicals works by inhibiting monoamine oxidase, an enzyme which helps regulate the function of the nervous system. This group is very useful in treating mites and ticks that are resistant to the traditional anticholinesterase insecticides. Amitraz is a common example of this class.

FORMULAS AND EXAMPLES[23]

To use wettable powders (WP), use the following formula to find the number of kilograms of wettable powder to mix in the spray tank.

$$\frac{A \times S}{W} = \text{amount of WP in kilograms}$$

Where: A = amount finished spray in liters
S = percent spray mix desired
W = % wettable powder

Example: To make 20 liters of a 0.06% spray mix from a 25% WP

$$\frac{20 \text{ liters} \times 0.06\% \text{ spray}}{25\% \text{ WP}} = 0.048 \text{ kg} = 48 \text{ gm. of WP}$$

To use an emulsifiable concentrate (EC), emulsifiable liquid insecticide (ELI), or water dispersible liquid (WDL,) use the following formula to find the number of liters to mix in the spray tank.

$$\frac{A \times S}{C} = \text{quantity of liquid in liters}$$

Where: A = amount finished spray in liters
S = percent spray mix desired
C = % concentration liquid product

Example: To make 100 liters of a 0.06% spray mix from a 12% EC

$$\frac{100 \text{ liters} \times 0.06\% \text{ spray}}{12\% \text{ EC}} = .5 \text{ liter of EC}$$

Other helpful conversions for liquids are:	Metric conversions:
1 gallon (gal.) = 4 quarts (qts.)	1 kg = 2.2 pounds
1 gallon = 128 fluid ounces (oz.)	30 mls. ~ 1 fluid ounce
1 quart = 2 pints (pts.)	500 mls. ~ 1 pint
1 pint = 16 ounces	1000 mls. ~ 1 quart
1 fluid ounce = 2 tablespoons (tbsp.)	4000 mls. ~ 1 gallon
1 tablespoon = 3 teaspoons (tsp.)	

Following are suggestions for treatments for specific pests. This information was condensed from the booklet produced by the Texas Agricultural Extension Service listed in the bibliography. These are general guidelines only. Listing all available products and directions is beyond the scope of this publication. **PLEASE READ AND FOLLOW DIRECTIONS ON THE LABEL OF THE SPECIFIC PRODUCT YOU ARE USING.**

BEEF CATTLE AND NON-LACTATING DAIRY CATTLE [23]

Cattle Grubs

Administer treatments between May and September 1, preferably soon after May 1 for best results. Animals should not be treated for grub control and internal parasites with certain products on the same day.

1. Dips	Coumaphos	25% WP Minimum number of days from last application until slaughter to prevent residue in meat 0. 42% flowable Do not apply to non-lactating dairy animals within 14 days of freshening (milking). Do not treat animals less than 3 months old. Do not treat sick or stressed stock. Also controls horn flies, lice and ticks.
	Phosmet	11.6% EC Minimum 21 days from last application to slaughter. Also controls horn flies.
2. Sprays	Note:	Thoroughly wet animals to the skin with spray from a high pressure sprayer using up to 1 gallon of finished formulation per animal.
	Coumaphos	25% WP Minimum 0 days to slaughter. 11.6% EC Same as for Coumaphos above. Do not spray animals for 10 days before or after shipping or weaning.
3. Pour-ons	Note:	Under certain conditions, some pour-ons may cause minor skin irritation and scaling.
	Famphur	13.2% EC Minimum 35 days to slaughter.

Use with caution on Brahman cattle. Do not use on dairy cows or within 21 days of freshening (milking). Also controls horn flies and aids in louse control.

	<u>Ivermectin</u>	1% ready to use Minimum 48 days to slaughter. Do not treat diary cattle of breeding age.
4. Spot-ons	<u>Fenthion</u>	20% Minimum 45 days to slaughter. Do not treat dairy cattle of breeding age. Do not treat within 10 days of dipping or weaning.
5. Injectables	<u>Ivermectin</u>	1% ready to use Minimum 35 days to slaughter.

Use subcutaneous injection only.

Horn Fly:	<u>Diazinon</u>	40% ear tag Minimum 0 days to slaughter. 20% ear tag Use 1-2 tags per animal when horn flies exceed 250-300 per animal.
	<u>Dischlorvos</u>	21.8% EC Minimum 0 days to slaughter.
	<u>Permethrin</u>	1% dust Minimum 0 days to slaughter. Install at proper height for maximum effectiveness.
	<u>Stirofos</u>	50% WP Minimum 0 days to slaughter. Use 1/2 to 1 gallon dilute spray per animal.

Ticks:	<u>Amitraz</u>	12.5% EC Minimum 0 days to slaughter. Use 1 quart in 100 gallons of water.

Lice:	Amitraz	12.5% EC Minimum 0 days to slaughter.
	Ivermectin	1% pour-on Minimum 48 days to slaughter. Do not treat dairy cattle of breeding age.
	Permethrin	1% pour-on Minimum 0 days to slaughter. Do not dilute. Apply 15 mls. per 45 kg. 0.25% dust Rub into coat; repeat for lice at 14 days.
Spinose Ear Tick:	Coumaphos	5% dust Minimum 0 days to slaughter.
	Fenvalerate	8% ear tag Minimum 0 days to slaughter. Use a tag in both ears.
	Permethrin	10% EC Minimum 0 days to slaughter. Apply 15 mls. oil or water mix per ear or 60-120 mls. per face or about a pint down backline.

Screw worm and Other Blow Fly Larvae:

Treat wounds and surrounding area thoroughly, but do not use excessive amounts. Treat twice the first week and weekly thereafter until healed.

Coumaphos	25% WP Minimum 0 days to slaughter. 11.6% EC 42% ELI Do not apply to dry dairy animals within 14 days of freshening.

Mange and Scab Mites:	Amitraz	12.5% EC	Minimum 0 days to slaughter. Two treatments 7-10 days apart are required for scabies mites.
	Lindane	10% EC	Minimum 30-60 days to slaughter. Can be used as a spray or dip.
	Permethrin	10% EC 11% EC 5.7% EC	Minimum 0 days to slaughter. Spray till soaked, repeat in 2-3 weeks.

LACTATING DAIRY CATTLE

Note: Certain materials may be used safely if they are applied correctly, but others are not recommended because they may contaminate the milk.

	Permethrin	10% EC	Minimum 0 days to slaughter. Use 2-4 liters of dilute spray per head; repeat in 14-21 days.
Horn Fly:	Coumaphos	1% dust	Minimum 0 days to slaughter.
	Methoxychlor	5% dust 50% WP	Minimum 0 days to slaughter. Do not use in conjunction with or following permethrin.
Stable Fly & House Fly:	Dichlorvos	21.8% EC	Minimum 0 days to slaughter. Do not exceed 60 mls. diluted spray mix per animal. Do not contaminate dairy feed.

Pyrethrins — 0.03% ready to use
Minimum 0 days to slaughter.

Apply enough spray to wet ends of hair but not hide.

Screwworm & Other Blow Fly Larvae: Treat wound and surrounding area twice the first week and then weekly until healed.

SHEEP AND NON-LACTATING GOATS

Lice, Ticks & Keds:

Coumaphos — 25% WP Minimum 0 days to slaughter.
0.125% EC

Use 0.06% spray or dip for lice or for ticks or keds. Do not use on lactating milk goats or dry animals within 14 days of freshening. Agitate dip before use.

5% dust For spot treatment application. (keds)

Lindane — 10% EC Minimum 30-60 days to slaughter.

Do not treat milk goats. Do not treat animals less than 3 months old.

Nose Bots: Invermectin — 0.08% drench Minimum 11 days to slaughter.

Apply 3 mls. per 12 kg. of body weight as an oral drench.

Fleeceworm or Wool Maggot:

Coumaphos — 25% WP Minimum 0 days to slaughter
Do not use on lactating dairy goats or dry animals within 14 days of freshening.

3% spray foam
or
5% dust For spot treatment application.

SWINE

Lice: Treat thoroughly. Do not treat for external parasites and vaccinate on the same day. Repeat application after 2-3 weeks.

Amitraz 12% EC Minimum 1 day to slaughter. Mix 500 mls. in 100 liters water.

Ivermectin 1% injectable Minimum 18 days to slaughter. Subcutaneously inject 1 ml. for each 34 kg. body weight.

Sarcoptic Mange Mite:

Amitraz 12.5% EC Minimum 1 day to slaughter Spray with coarse nozzle; mix 500 ml. in 100 liters water.

Fenvalerate 10% WDL Minimum 1 day to slaughter Wet animals thoroughly; repeat at 14 day intervals.

HORSES

Bots: Dichlorvos 17.5% liquid Check label for use restrictions.

Ivermectin 1.87% oral paste Follow label instructions.

Trichlorfon 40% oral paste Do not treat foals less than 4 months old or mares in last month of pregnancy.

Lice, Horn Fly, Stable Fly, Ticks & Mosquitoes:

Coumaphos	0.06-0.125% Spray	Do not treat animal less than 3 months old. Do not use with oral drenches or other internal parasite medications or with pyrethroids or their synergists or other organophosphates. Repeat as necessary.
	1% dust (horn fly)	Dust lightly in ears for ticks.
	5% dust	For screwworms, treat wound thoroughly.
	3% spray	Cover thoroughly. Spray wound.
Permethrin	10% EC	Wet horse thoroughly.
	5% wipe-on	Sponge animal thoroughly with 2 liters of mix.

POULTRY

House Fly & Soldier Fly:

Carbaryl	5% dust or	Minimum 7 days to slaughter.
	50% WP	Use either 2.2 kg. of 5% dust or 37.3 mg of 50% wp in 4 liters water per 100 birds. Bird treatment is used as a supplement to roost and building treatment.
Permethrin	10% EC	Minimum 0 days to slaughter. Use 30-60 ml. per bird; cover vent thoroughly.
Stirofos	50% WP	Minimum 0 days to slaughter.

			Spray birds lightly while treating litter surface. Repeat as necessary, but not more often than every 14 days.
Fowl Tick:	Carbaryl	50% WP	Treat roosts and buildings only.
	Stirofos	50% WP	Minimum 0 days to slaughter. Apply a 1% spray to walls, ceiling, floor cracks.
Chiggers:	Chlorpyrifos	25% WP	Do not apply directly to turkeys. Spray a 3-5 meter protective area around turkey pens with a 0.59% spray.
Depluming Mite:			
	Sulfur Dust		Use 11-22 kg. of elemental sulfur per area.

Premises Treatment

Inside and outside of animal quarters

Note:	Avoid direct application to exposed feed and water. Do not use where milk is processed. Do not use during milking time when milk and utensils may become contaminated.		
	Dichlorvos	21.8% EC	Direct 0.5-1.0% mist over entire area where flies congregate.
	Fenvalerate	10% WDL	Apply to fly resting areas.
	Permethrin	11% EC 25% WP 10% EC, and others	Apply to fly resting areas.

SECTION **10**

INJECTABLE SEDATIVES, TRANQUILIZERS, ANALGESICS AND ANESTHETICS

INJECTABLE SEDATIVES, TRANQUILIZERS, ANALGESICS AND ANESTHETICS

Animals given tranquilizers and sedatives become calmer and less reactive to noises, movement and pain. Tranquilizers and sedatives are used before painful procedures such as surgery or before handling or examining difficult patients. In these situations the calming effects of the tranquilizer or sedative make the animal safer to handle.

Analgesics are drugs which relieve pain.

Anesthetics fall into two categories: local and general. Local anesthetics are injected around the desired area or into the nerve that supplies the desired area. Local anesthetics prevent the nerves from feeling pain. A general anesthetic works on the brain. An animal under a general anesthetic will appear to be asleep to the extent that it cannot be awakened. The animal given a general anesthetic will not move when a painful procedure is performed on it. General anesthetics are used most often to perform major surgery.

I. TRANQUILIZERS AND SEDATIVES

A. General Uses

1. To quiet an unruly animal for examination or for collecting samples for making a diagnosis.
2. Can be given along with local anesthetics in order to perform some surgeries.
3. May be used before general anesthesia to keep the animal calm as it goes to sleep and also as it wakes up.

B. Limitations

1. If the animal is depressed or very sick, the tranquilizer may affect the animal more than usual. Many of these drugs are broken down by the liver before the animal can awaken. If the liver is not working well, it will take longer for the animal to awaken. A smaller dose may be given to help lessen the effects.

2. If the animal is highly excited before the tranquilizer is given, the animal may become even more excited or the tranquilizer may have no effect at all.

3. If the tranquilizer is given to do a physical exam, it may affect the exam. Careful observation at a distance before giving the tranquilizer will help make the physical exam more accurate.

C. Drugs Used as Tranquilizers

1. Alpha-2 agonist tranquilizers.
   a) xylazine hydrochloride

    b) detomidine hydrochloride
    c) can reverse effects with yohimbine
2. Benzodiazepine tranquilizers.
    a) diazepam
    b) zolazepam
3. Buterophenone tranquilizers.
    a) azaperone
4. Phenothiazine tranquilizers.
    a) acepromazine maleate
    b) chlorpromazine hydrochloride

Alpha-2 Agonists

Indications: Sedation with analgesia.

Precautions: Causes the heart to slow and skip beats, therefore do not use in animals with a heart problem.

Use care when working around legs of horses because they may move quickly if surprised or hurt.

DO NOT USE IN PREGNANT COWS OR SHEEP IN THE LAST THIRD OF PREGNANCY AS IT MAY CAUSE ABORTIONS.

Safety - low doses produce the same effects in people.

DETOMIDINE

Indications: More potent than xylazine. Safer to work around the legs of horses given detomidine compared to those given xylazine. Effective in excited animals. Used for standing restraint in animals and as an analgesic for belly pain.

Dosage and Route:

Horse - 20-40 micrograms/kg IV or IM

Maximum effect 5-10 minutes, 30-45 minute duration.

When given before ketamine for general anesthesia, 22-44 micrograms/kg.

Cow - 10-20 micrograms/kg IV

20-40 micrograms/kg IM

Sedation in 15-20 minutes, lasting up to 1 hour.

Sheep - 10 micrograms/kg IV

Lasts 20-120 minutes after being given.

XYLAZINE

Indications: Less expensive and less potent than detomidine.

Precautions: DO NOT USE ALONE IF WORKING AROUND THE BACK LEGS IN HORSES.

DO NOT USE IF ANIMAL HAS HEART PROBLEMS, ESPECIALLY SKIPPING BEATS.
DO NOT USE IN LATE PREGNANCY IN COWS, SHEEP, OR GOATS AS IT MAY CAUSE ABORTIONS.
DO NOT USE IN CATS.

Dosage and Route: Sedation 3-5 minutes after IV dose, 10-15 minutes after IM administration, lasts 1-2 hours; analgesia lasts 15-30 minutes. May be reversed using yohimbine.

Horse - Standing sedation 0.44-0.55 mg/kg IV. 0.88-1.1 mg/kgIM.
For preanesthetic before ketamine or Telazol 1.1 mg/kgIV
Preanesthetic to all other combinations 0.33-0.66 mg/kgIV
Yohimbine reversal- 0.075 mg/kg IV[15]

Foals - 0.44-0.55 mg/kg IV. 0.88-1.1 mg/kg IM.

Cows - 0.055-0.11 mg/kg IV. 0.11-0.22 mg/kg IM.
Note: This dose will cause the cow to lie down. Give lower doses if standing
tranquilization is desired. DO NOT GIVE IN LATE PREGNANCY.
Yohimbine reversal- 0.125 mg/kg[15]

Sheep - 0.05-0.1 mg/kg IV. 0.1-0.2 mg/kg IM.
Note: Sheep are less sensitive to xylazine than cattle.
Yohimbine reversal- 0.125 mg/kg IV[15]

Goats - 0.05- 0.075 mg/kg IV. 0.1-0.15 mg/kg IM.
Note: Goats are more sensitive to xylazine than cattle.
Yohimbine reversal- 0.125 mg/kg[15]

Pigs - 1.65 mg/kg IV. 2.2 mg/kg IM.
Note: Not reliably effective in pigs.

Llamas[17]- 0.1-0.25 mg/kg SQ or IV before ketamine or alone
Yohimbine reversal- 0.125 mg/kg IV[15]

Guinea Pigs[18] - 5 mg/kg IM with ketamine at 20-40 mg/kg mixed in the same syringe.
Lasts 15-35 minutes.

Rabbits[19]- 1.0-3.0 mg/kg IV. 4.0-5.0 mg/kg IM.

Birds- Do not give xylazine alone- combine with ketamine.
Safer IV than IM.
DO NOT GIVE TO A BIRD WITH KIDNEY OR LIVER DISEASE.
Give 10-30 mg/kg ketamine combined with 2-6 mg/kg xylazine combined in the same syringe.

XYLAZINE COMBINATIONS

a) <u>xylazine/acepromazine</u>

Horses[16] - Safer to work around legs than with xylazine alone.

0.044 mg/kg acepromazine IV with 0.44 mg/kg xylazine IV at the same time in the same syringe, or give the xylazine 10 minutes after the acepromazine.

b) <u>xylazine/butorphanol</u>

Combination gives increased analgesia.

Horses - standing restraint 0.1-0.5 mg/kg xylazine IV, followed in 5 minutes with butorphanol 0.01-0.04 mg/kg IV

Cows - Xylazine 0.01-0.02 mg/kg IV + butorphanol 0.01-0.02 mg/kg IV at the same time in the same syringe for standing restraint. To lay down - 0.05-0.1 mg/kg xylazine IV and 0.01-0.02 mg/kgbutorphanol IV.

c) <u>detomidine/butorphanol</u>

Horses - 10.0 micrograms/kg detomidine IV with 0.05 mg/kg butorphanol IV

<u>Benzodiazepine Tranquilizers</u>

<u>Indications</u>: Decreases anxiety. Useful to stop seizure activity. Very little ill effects on the heart or lungs, therefore safer for old or sick animals. Relaxes muscles.

<u>Contraindications</u>: May take longer to recover if liver is not working well.

DIAZEPAM

Horse - 0.02-0.1 mg/kg IV for sedation

Note: Give injection slowly because rapid injection may cause excitement.

For seizure prevention, 0.1-0.15 mg/kg IV.

For seizure prevention in newborn foals, 0.11-0.44 mg/kg IV.

Cow - Give 0.4 mg/kg slowly into the vein for brief (5-10 minutes) of sedation with laying down; full recovery occurs in 45-60 minutes.

Sheep and Goats - 0.11 mg/kg IV when given with ketamine for general anesthesia.

0.25-0.5 mg/kg IV for sedation[16].

Swine - Because of the high doses required in pigs, diazepam is not generally used.

ZOLAZEPAM

More potent than diazepam.

Is used only in combination with tiletamine to provide general anesthesia.

Buterophenone Tranquilizers

AZAPERONE

Indications: Made for use in pigs-will usually make the pig lie down. Animal can still be aroused by pain. May be used to calm a nervous sow or gilt after having piglets. May cause a short time of excitement after giving IM.

PRECAUTIONS: DO NOT GIVE TO ANIMALS IN SHOCK. USE A LOWER DOSE IN OLD OR ANEMIC ANIMALS.

Dosage and Route:

Pigs - 0.5-2.2 mg/kg IM. Use lower dose for mild sedation. More than 2.2 mg/kg will make the animal lie down. Do not give more than 1.0 mg/kg in mature boars.

Phenothiazine Tranquilizers

Indications: Sedation in animals

PRECAUTIONS: DO NOT USE IN ANIMALS IN SHOCK. USE A LOWER DOSE IN OLD ANIMALS OR ANEMIC ANIMALS. MAY INCREASE EXCITEMENT IF GIVEN TO AN ANIMAL THAT IS ALREADY EXCITED. DO NOT GIVE TO ANIMALS HAVING SEIZURES OR A HISTORY OF SEIZURES. DO NOT GIVE TO MALES HAVING PENILE PROBLEMS, ESPECIALLY STALLIONS. DO NOT GIVE TO ANIMALS THAT HAVE RECENTLY BEEN DEWORMED WITH AN ORGANOPHOSPHATE DEWORMER.

CHLORPROMAZINE HYDROCHLORIDE

Indications: Used more in small animals than large animals.

Dosage and Route:

Horse[16] - 1.1-2.2 mg/kg IV or IM
IV: effective 5-15 minutes after being given, lasts 5-8 hours.
IM: effective after 45-60 minutes, lasts 12-18 hours.

Cattle[16] - 0.2-1.1 mg/kg IV. 1.1-2.2 mg/kg IM.

Sheep and Goats - 0.55- 4.4 mg/kg IV or 2.2-6.6 mg/kg IM

Pigs - 1.1 mg/kg IM

Dogs[15] - 0.11 mg/kg to stop vomiting. 1-2 mg/kg to tranquilize IM or IV, lasts 8 hours.

Cats - 1 mg/kg IM

ACEPROMAZINE MALEATE

Onset of action 15-20 minutes after IV injection, lasts 2 hours.

Horse[16] - 0.044-0.088 mg/kg IV or IM

Cows - 0.01-0.02 mg/kg IV or IM

Goats and Sheep - if weigh less than 50 kg, 0.1 0.2 mg/kg IV. If weigh more than 50 kg, 0.05-0.01 mg/kg IV.

Pigs - 0.11-0.44 mg/kg IV or IM, to a maximum of 15 mg.

Dogs[15] - 0.062-0.25 mg/kg IV, IM, or SQ. Maximum IV dose 3 mg. May be given by mouth at 1.1-2.2 mg/kg.

Cats[15] - 0.062-0.25 mg/kg IV, IM, or SQ. Maximum IV dose 1 mg. May be given by mouth at 1.1-2.2 mg/kg.

II. ANALGESICS

A. General Uses

1. To relieve pain in an animal.
2. Non-steroidal antiinflammatories can lower fevers.

B. Limitations

1. If the animal is dehydrated or in shock, the non-steroidal antiinflammatories may cause damage to the kidneys.
2. Non-steroidal antiinflammatories may cause stomach ulcers. Very young animals are especially susceptible. Indicators of ulcers are inappetence, vomiting and dark brown to black, tar-like, feces.
3. Non-steroidal antiinflammatories can slow blood clotting.
4. Steroidal antiinflammatories make the immune system less able to fight disease.
5. Opioid analgesics may cause the gut to stop working and makes the animal breathe less deeply.

C. Drugs used as analgesics.

1. Non-opiate/opioid analgesic agents

a) alpha-2 agonists (note: these drugs are also tranquilizers; dosages are listed under tranquilizers)

i) xylazine - up to 100 minutes pain relief in gut, 35-40 minutes in rest of body

ii) detomidine - up to 4 hours pain relief in gut, 2 hours in rest of body

b) Non-steroidal anti-inflammatory drugs- mild analgesia without sedation

i) phenylbutazone

Horse[16] 2-4 mg/kg IV every 12 hrs

Note: If injection is given around the vein instead of in the vein, severe damage and loss of tissue will result.[15] or 2.2-4.4 mg/kg into mouth once daily[15]
Note: May cause ulcers in the mouth if held between the cheek and gums.

Cows[15] - 4 mg/kg IV or PO every other day

Pigs - 4 mg/ kg IV or PO daily

Dogs- 15 mg/ kg four times a day or 22 mg/kg three times a day PO; give no more than 800 mg per day.
Llamas[15] - 2.2-4.4 mg/kg IV or PO daily

ii) flunixin meglumine

Indications: Works well for relieving belly pain, lowering fevers and helping counteract the poisons of some bacteria.
Horse - 1.1 mg/kg IV or IM every 12 hours
Note: May get severe infection in the muscle when given IM. Use penicillin if the horse becomes infected in an injection spot. In young horses use one or two doses **only** as it may cause stomach ulcers.
Cow[15] - 1.1 mg/kg IV or IM. Give every other day.
Note: May cause stomach ulcers in young calves.
Llama[15]- 1.1 mg/kg IV or IM once daily

iii) dipyrone

Indications: Dipyrone is most effective at lowering fevers. It is less effective at relieving pain.
Horse[16]- 11 mg/kg IV or IM every 8 to 12 hours as needed
Cow[15]- 2.5-10 grams every 8 to 12 hours as needed
Llama[15]- 11 mg/kg IV or IM every 8-12 hours as needed
Sheep and Pigs - 2.5 grams every 8-12 hours as needed
Dogs and Cats - 27.5 mg/kg every 8-12 hours as needed

iv) aspirin

Indications: Aspirin is potent as an anti-inflammatory drug. In horses with long term inflammation in the eye aspirin is commonly used.
Precautions:
DO NOT GIVE TO AN ANIMAL THAT IS DEHYDRATED.
DO NOT GIVE TO AN ANIMAL THAT IS BLEEDING OR IN SHOCK.
DO NOT GIVE TO AN ANIMAL ON WHICH SURGERY IS TO BE DONE.
DISCONTINUE TREATMENT IF THE ANIMAL SHOWS SYMPTOMS OF STOMACH ULCERS.
Horse[15]- 25 mg/kg twice the first day, than 30 mg/kg once daily.
Cows and Sheep - 100 mg/kg every 12 hours
Swine[15] - 10 mg/kg every 6 hours
Dogs[15]- 25-35 mg/kg every 12 hours for joint pain.

10 mg/kg every 12 hours for other pain relief and to lower fever.

Cats[15]- 10 mg/kg every 48 hours (TOXIC IF GIVEN MORE OFTEN).

2. Opiate/opioid analgesics

These drugs have potential to be abused by people so closely regulate the amount dispensed and the need for refills.

a) sedation and analgesia

i) butorphanol

Butorphanol is best used in combination with a tranquilizer since excitement can occur if it is used alone. See dosage combinations under tranquilizers.

ii) pentazocine

Horse[16] 0.44-0.88 mg/kg IV or IM

May be used in cases of colic (gut pain).

Has a similar potency to butorphanol, but does not last as long.

b) antagonists- these drugs reverse the effects of certain opiates.

i) naloxone

Horse[16] 9.9 micrograms/kg IV

III. ANESTHETICS

A. General Uses

1. Anesthetics are required to perform surgery, some obstetrical procedures, and some special diagnostic procedures, and to apply casts and splints.
2. Anesthetics may be used when it would be dangerous for the animal to move during a procedure or for the operator to perform the procedure.

B. Types of Anesthesia

1. General Anesthesia (animal is unconscious)

a) Advantages

-no movement

-good for short surgery

Disadvantages

-in a sick animal can cause death

-have to wait for animal to break down drug to wake up unless a reversal drug exists

-animal may hurt itself if it tries to stand too soon

-animal's body may be damaged if kept under anesthetic too long

b) drugs used

i) barbiturates

Indications: Short anesthetic for a quick procedure where complete anesthesia is needed.

Contraindications:

The liver has to breakdown the barbiturate for the animal to wake up, therefore do not use in animals if the liver or kidneys are not working.

If the animal is shocky, do not use.

In animals that are less than 1 month old or extremely old, do not use.

In extremely thin animals, do not use.

DO NOT USE IN SIGHT HOUNDS.

a. Oxybarbiturates- difficult to use in large animals

i. Pentobarbital- used for surgery, to control seizures, sedation.

Decrease the amount of pentobarbital given if the animal has received analgesics or tranquilizers. 88 mg/kg will kill any animal.

Horses[16]- 26.0 mg/kg IV

Half of the dose is injected as a rapid bolus to prevent the excitable phase.

The remainder may be given to effect.

Cows, Sheep, and Goats[16] - same as the horse

Pigs[16] - same as the horse or the entire calculated dose may be given into the belly cavity.

Dogs and Cats[15] 25-30 mg/kg IV for anesthesia

ii. Methohexital - do not use in large animal anesthesia because animals undergo violent recoveries.

b. Thiobarbiturates

i. Thiopental sodium

Needs refrigeration after solution is mixed if it is not used immediately.

Repeated doses of thiopental will saturate tissues, the animal will have to break down the drug to wake up.

Decreases lung function and respiratory rate.

Horse[16] - After tranquilizer, use 6.6-8.8 mg/kg as a 5-10% solution given rapidly IV. Control the horses head as the thiopental is given as the horse will back up and could flip over backwards. Up to 5.0 grams total dose may be given to an adult horse to keep it under. A tranquilizer usually is needed to help calm the recovering horse. Thiopental may be combined with guaifenesin solutions, which is a muscle relaxant, and given IV rapidly to lay an animal down.

Cow[16] - 6.6-8.8 mg/kg IV in an unsedated animal.
Decrease the dose if the animal is sedated.

Sheep and Goats[16] 6.6-11.0 mg/kg IV in unsedated animals.
Decrease the dose if the animal is sedated.

Llamas[17] - 8.8-11 mg/kg IV

Rabbits[19] - 30-45 mg/kg IV slowly

ii. Thiamylal sodium

Not being made in the US at this time.

May be given IV mixed in solution with guaifenesin, a muscle relaxant.

Horse[16] - 10.0 mg/kg in unsedated horses.
Decrease the dose if the horse is sedated.
Can show excitement when recovering- make sure an animal handler can steady the horse by controlling the head.

Cow[16] - 6.6-8.8 mg/kg IV in unsedated animals.
Decrease the dose if the animal is sedated.

Sheep and Goats[16] - 6.6-11.0 mg/kg in unsedated animals.
Decrease the dose if the animal is sedated.

Pigs[16] - 6.6-11.0 mg/kg IV in unsedated animals.
Decrease the dose if the animals are sedated.

ii) non-barbiturates

a. chloral hydrate

The dose for anesthesia is very close to the dose that kills. Chloral hydrate is safer when used with pentobarbital and magnesium sulfate. It can be used for standing procedures.

DO NOT GIVE TO ANIMALS WITH LIVER OR KIDNEY PROBLEMS.

DO NOT GIVE TO ANIMALS LESS THAN 1 MONTH OLD.

DO NOT ADMINISTER AS A SOLUTION STRONGER THAN 7 PERCENT CHLORAL HYDRATE IV.

Horse[16] - 88.0-110.0 mg/kg slowly IV to effect.

May give up to 220.0 mg/kg IV when used alone in unsedated horses.

Cows[16] - 88.0-110.0 mg/kg slowly IV to effect, up to 220.0 mg/kg.

Pigs[16] - 245.0 mg/kg or 3.5 ml/kg of 7 percent solution IV to effect.

b. ketamine hydrochloride

Works best when combined with a tranquilizer.

May have poor muscle relaxation.

Can increase pressure inside the eye.

Can increase the likelihood of seizures.

Do not use if animal has liver or kidney disease.

Horse[16] - DO NOT GIVE KETAMINE IF THE ANIMAL IS NOT RESPONDING TO THE TRANQUILIZER.

*Tranquilize with xylazine 1.1 mg/kg IV. When the horses head is level with its knees (about 5 minutes) give 1.76-2.2 mg/kg ketamine IV. Gives 5-10 minutes of anesthesia and 10-20 minutes of being down.

*Tranquilize with 0.22-0.33 mg/kg diazepam IM. After 20 minutes, give above dose of xylazine + ketamine combined in the same syringe IV. Gives 20-25 minutes of anesthesia and 30-40 minutes of being down.

*Tranquilize with 22 micrograms/kg detomidine IV. Wait 6-10 minutes, then give 2.2 mg/kg ketamine IV. Anesthesia may last as long as 25 minutes. Do not give the ketamine if the animal does not become tranquil from the detomidine.

*One gram of ketamine can be combined with 1 liter of 5% guaifenesin or 500 ml of 10% guaifenesin. Tranquilize with xylazine, acepromazine or detomidine. After tranquilized, give the solution rapidly IV to produce recumbency. Slow the drip to maintain recumbency.

*Combine 5% guaifenesin (50 mg/ml), 0.05% xylazine (0.5 mg/ml) and 1.0-2.0 mg/ml ketamine. The solution can be given rapidly IV to induce anesthesia in foals, then used to maintain anesthesia by slowing the drip. In adult horses anesthesia can be started using the above doses of xylazine-ketamine, then maintain anesthesia dripping 2-3 ml/kg/hr into the vein. If greater than 2-3 ml/kg/hr is needed to keep the horse under anesthesia, decrease the ketamine to 1.0 mg/ml or decrease the xylazine to 0.25 mg/ml.

Cow[16]

*Tranquilize calves using xylazine at 0.1-0.2 mg/kg IM followed by Ketamine at10.0-15.0 mg/kg IM. Anesthesia lasts about 45 minutes. If more time is needed 3.0-5.0 mg/kg ketamine may be given IM. Adult cattle can be anesthetized with xylazine 0.1-0.2 mg/kg IV, followed by ketamine at 2.0 mg/kg IV. The combination should last about 30 minutes. If more time is needed, 15 more minutes can be obtained by giving 0.75-1.25 mg/kg IV.

*Diazepam at 0.11 mg/kg mixed in the same syringe with 4.4 mg/kg IV ketamine can be used to provide anesthesia for 10-15 minutes and recumbency for 20-30 minutes.

*A mixture of 5% guaifenesin (50 mg/ml), 0.1% ketamine (1 mg/ml) and 0.01% xylazine (0.1 mg/ml) may be given IV at 0.5 ml/kg to induce anesthesia, then 1.5 ml/kg/hr to maintain anesthesia in calves and 2.0 ml/kg/hr in adults to maintain anesthesia. If more than 2.0 ml/kg are needed to finish the procedure, decrease the amount of xylazine to 0.005% (0.05 mg/ml) to avoid a prolonged recovery because of the xylazine.

c. **tiletamine-zolazepam (Telazol)** - Refer to clinical technique sections for use in horses, cattle, sheep and goats and swine.

Llama[17]

0.5 - 2 mg/kg to effect, depending on the condition of the animal and the degree of sedation required.

c) drugs used to assist in general anesthesia

i) Anticholinergics

a) decreases some side effects of anesthetics. Helps to keep the heart rate normal, decreases saliva production, and slows gut motility.

b) atropine- not routinely used in large animals

c) glycopyrrolate

Horse and Swine - 0.005 mg/kg IV, IM, or SQ

Cow, Goat, or Sheep - 0.005-0.01 mg/kg IV, IM, or SQ

Note: Use with caution since the decrease in gut motility may cause colic.

ii) Muscle relaxants

a) smoooths induction and maintenance of anesthesia. Decreases the amount of anesthetic needed.

b) **guaifenesin** - refer to clinical technique sections for use.

2. Local Anesthesia

Animal is fully awake or may be tranquilized for a minor surgical procedure

Advantages

-safer for sick or weak animals

-good for diagnosing lameness

-not expensive

-minimal equipment required

Disadvantages

-may move during the procedure, which could cause injury to the animal or operator

-local or whole body reactions to anesthetic agents can occur

-some species will not tolerate certain techniques

-need additional restraint in most cases

a) Regional anesthesia

Blocks the pain impulses at a major nerve trunk. The major nerve supplies smaller nerves to a region of the body. For example the spinal cord is the major nerve trunk which is affected in an epidural block. Regional anesthesia usually prevents muscle movement in that region of the body the major nerve supplies and pain sensation from that region.

Agents used in regional anesthesia are most often either 2% lidocaine hydrochloride or 2% mepivicaine hydrochloride. The mepivicaine tends to have a longer duration, works more quickly, and causes less tissue reaction.

1. <u>Inverted L block.</u> This is the simplest form of regional anesthesia/analgesia. A line of anesthetic is injected just below the transverse processes of the lumbar vertebrae and another line of anesthetic just behind the last rib. No nerves entering the flank region are able to carry impulses of pain back to the brain. An 18-gauge needle, 3-5 cm long is used. The anesthetic should be injected into the full depth of the muscle wall. As much as 100 ml of local anesthetic may be used in cattle, and surgery should not begin until 10-15 minutes after injection. Sheep and goats are more susceptible to toxicity from too much lidocaine. Flank laparotomy may also be performed in the horse using the inverted L block.

INVERTED L BLOCK

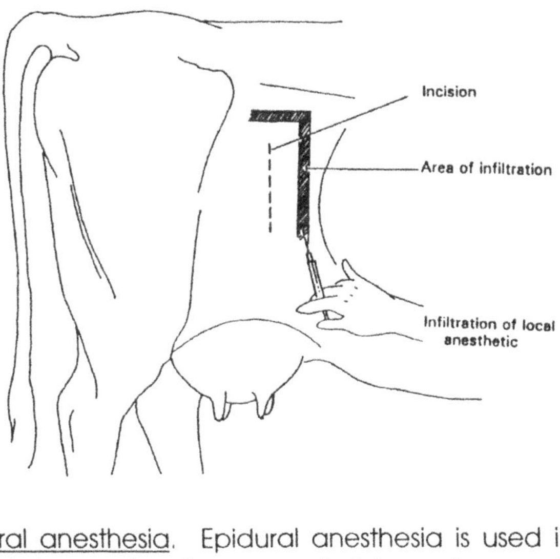

2. <u>Epidural anesthesia.</u> Epidural anesthesia is used in cattle and horses to decrease straining when assisting in delivering a baby or when returning a prolapsed vagina or uterus to its normal position. Surgery on the anus or vulva may be performed while the animal is under an epidural. Less commonly, epidurals may also be used in dogs, cats, sheep and goats. In cows the space to inject is between the first and second tail vertebrae. If the tail is grasped and moved up and down, the first obvious joint

is the spot to insert the needle. After clipping and scrubbing the spot, an 18-gauge 3-5 cm needle is inserted at a 45-degree angle until the progress is stopped. When the needle is in the correct location bubbles should appear in the syringe when aspirating and the anesthetic should inject easily. If blood is aspirated, the needle must be repositioned. The dosage of anesthetic is 0.5-1.0 ml per 50 kg of body weight. The lower dosage should be used first. If too much anesthetic is injected the animal will go down and may begin to have trouble breathing. A horse would become very agitated if its hindlegs quit working since they get up using their front legs first. A cow will lay down, since they get up using their hindlegs first.

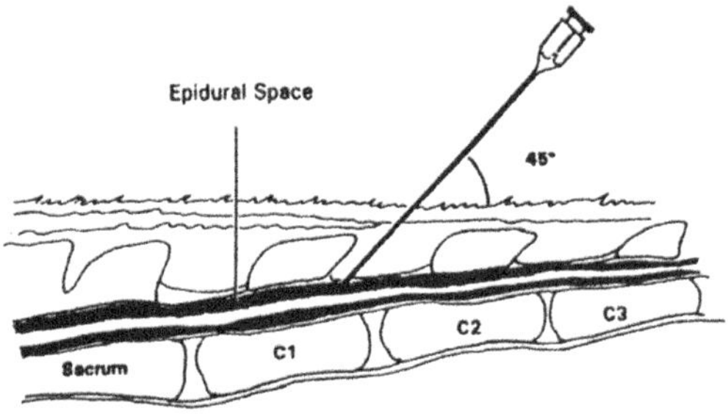

BOVINE EPIDURAL ANESTHESIA

Epidural anesthesia in the horse is performed by inserting the 18-gauge 3-5 cm needle through the space between the first and second tail vertebrae. In the horse this space is just above where the long tail hairs come out and is the first joint when moving the tail up and down. The needle is inserted at an angle of 30 degrees or 60 degrees and left in place. The area must be clipped and scrubbed before

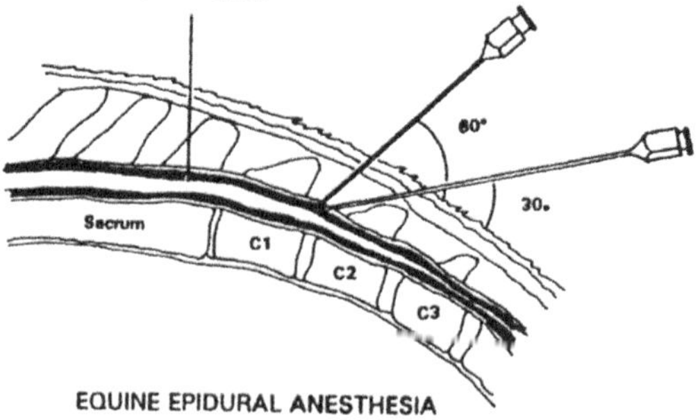

EQUINE EPIDURAL ANESTHESIA

inserting the needle. Five to 10 ml of anesthetic should be injected, starting with the lower dose first.

3. Intravenous limb anesthesia. For operations on the distal limb, especially in cattle, a tourniquet may be applied to the lower limb. A vein on the dorsal surface of the limb is located and 10-20 ml of local anesthetic injected into the vein. After the injection the area is massaged to prevent hematoma formation. The limb will be anesthetized after 5-10 minutes and will remain anesthetized for 1-2 hours as long as the tourniquet remains in place. After surgery the tourniquet should be removed slowly. A pad may be placed under the tourniquet to protect the limb while the tourniquet is in place.

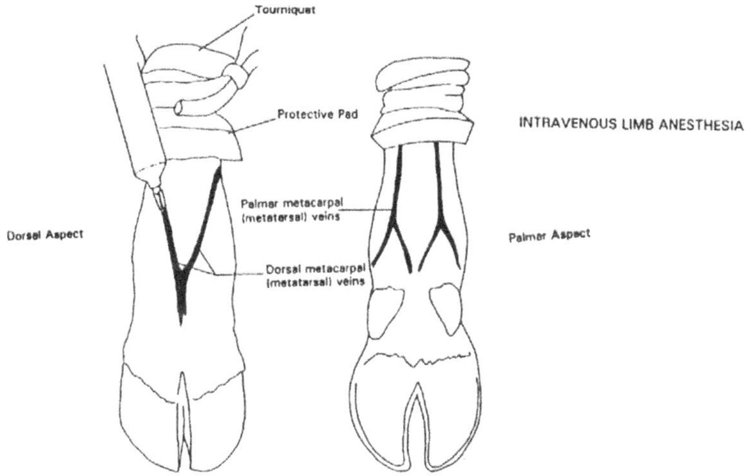

4. Nerve blocks in horses may be done over specific nerves in the horses limb. A ring block, encircling the limb, will anesthetize all of the limb below the level of the block. Nerve blocks may be used to perform a surgery or may be used to localize a lameness. LOCAL ANESTHETICS CONTAINING EPINEPHRINE SHOULD NEVER BE USED IN THE HORSE. The epinephrine causes the muscle in the blood vessel walls to contract and can cut off circulation to the end of the limb. Horses are more sensitive to this effect than other animals.

Palmar digital nerve block. Two mls of local anesthetic injected over the small cord-like palmar digital nerve halfway between the fetlock and the hoof on the lateral and medial side of the limb will anesthetize the heel and back third of the foot. The area should be scrubbed but does not have to be clipped.

Abaxial sesamoid block. At the sides of the sesamoid bones in the fetlock the palmar digital nerve can be rolled under the finger. Two mls of anesthetic can be injected over the nerve. The area should be cleaned but does not need to be clipped. A 25-gauge needle causes less reaction from the horse. This block, about 5 minutes after injection, anesthetizes the pastern and coffin areas. There may be a small area on the front of the hoof that would not be blocked.

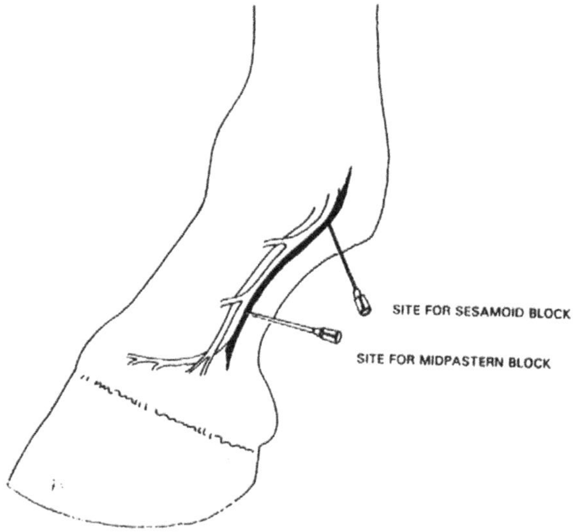

b) Local anesthetic infilltrated at the surgical site.

This anesthetizes the small nerves which enter muscle or skin. The drawback of its use in this manner is some distortion of tissue at the site of the surgery.

Clinical Techniques In Equine Anesthesia[16]

General considerations:

Preanesthetic tranquilization should always be used in horses unless their condition contraindicates it.

I. Tranquilizers and sedatives

A. Acepromazine -- 0.044 mg/kg IV given 20-30 minutes prior to anesthesia.

B. Alpha-2 agents

These are given IV 5 minutes prior to induction with ketamine or Telazol®. They are given IV 10-15 minutes prior to induction with other agents. They can be given IM 15-20 minutes prior to induction.

1. Xylazine given at 0.33-0.66 mg/kg IV or 1.1 mg/kg IM. It is given at 1.1 mg/kg if ketamine or Telazol® is being used.
2. Detomidine is given at 5.0-10.0 microgram/kg IV. It is given at 22.0 microgram/kg IV if ketamine or Telazol® is being used as induction agent.

II. Induction of anesthesia

A. Thiobarbiturates such as thiamylal or thiopental in a 5% solution can be given rapidly IV at 6.6-8.8 mg/kg. Some horses back up and may even flip over backwards as the drug affects them so handle them accordingly. Thiobarbiturates must be given IV or massive tissue damage will occur. This amount of drug will give 10-15 minutes of anesthesia.

B. Ketamine

1. With xylazine. After xylazine has exerted its effect, ketamine is administered at 1.76-2.2 mg/kg IV. Usually after 1-2 minutes the horse lays down. This combination gives about 10 minutes of anesthesia and 15-20 minutes before the horse is ready to stand up. Do not administer ketamine if 1-2 injections of xylazine does not provide tranquilization. If excess ketamine has been given or if the horse is experiencing a violent recovery, more xylazine at 0.22-0.44 mg/kg IV should be given. Ketamine does not always induce anesthesia in excited horses.
2. With xylazine and diazepam. After xylazine has exerted its effect, diazepam is given at 0.022-0.033 mg/kg IV along

with ketamine at 2.2 mg/kg IV. The diazepam and ketamine can be mixed in the same syringe. Duration of anesthesia is the same as above, but the anesthetic control is improved. An alternative regimen uses xylazine at 0.3 mg/kg IV followed by diazepam at 0.1 mg/kg IV and ketamine at 2.2 mg/kg IV. For anesthesia of 20-25 minutes and recumbency of 30-40 minutes give diazepam at 0.22 mg/kg IM 20 minutes before giving xylazine at I.I mg/kg IV. After 5 minutes give ketamine at 2.2 mg/kg IV.

3. With xylazine and butorphanol. Butorphanol at 0.044 mg/kg IV is given at the same time as the xylazine. The ketamine is given at 2.2 mg/kg IV after the horse has become tranquil. Duration of recumbency is 20-25 minutes.
4. With detomidine. After the horse has become tranquil from the detomidine give ketamine at 2.2 mg/kg IV. Usually the horse will lay down within 1-2 minutes. This combination gives 15 minutes of anesthesia and 20-25 minutes of recumbency. If the horse is not affected from 1-2 injections of detomidine then ketamine should not be given. Compared to xylazine-ketamine, when horses stand they remain wobbly for a longer period of time.

C. Guaifenesin

1. Guaifenesin must be given by rapid intravenous administration for proper induction. As a 5% (50 gm/L) solution it is given to effect through a 12-gauge catheter or needle in adults and 14 to 16-gauge in foals. If a solution of 7 or 10% is used a slightly smaller needle or catheter can be used. Also, inflammation of the vein should be expected with the stronger solutions. A person handling the horse's head and tail are needed for the horse will go down in an uncontrolled manner. The dose to induce recumbency is 110.0 mg/kg. Overdoses occur when 2.5-3 times this amount is given and is seen as straightening and stiffening of the limbs. IT IS BEST NOT TO USE GUAIFENESIN ALONE FOR ANESTHESIA BECAUSE OF THE LARGE VOLUME OF DRUG NEEDED TO INDUCE RECUMBENCY AND ITS LACK OF ANALGESIA.
2. With thiobarbiturate. Add 2 gm (3 gm for horses greater than 500 kg) of thiamylal or thiopental to one liter of 5% guaifenesin (or 500 ml of 10% guaifenesin) and administer rapidly IV The dose is 110.0 mg/kg. Animals usually will become recumbent after 75% of the dose is given and if no more is administered, 10-15 minutes of anesthesia is

provided. An alternate method involves giving guaifenesin to about 55 mg/kg, then completing the induction with the thiobarbiturate at 3.3-4.4 mg/kg in one quick injection.

3. With ketamine. Add 1.0 gm (2.2 mg/kg for horses greater than 500 kg) to a liter of 5% or 500 ml of 10% guaifenesin. The dose is 110.0 mg/kg. 10-15 minutes of anesthesia is provided when recumbency is reached (75% of calculated dose is given). An alternate method involves giving guaifenesin to about 55 mg/kg, then completing induction by injecting ketamine at 1.3-1.75 mg/kg. With this method xylazine (0.3-0.5 mg/kg IV) should be given prior to the guaifenesin.

D. Telazol®

1. Telazol® should not be used alone for anesthesia because of poor muscle relaxation and excitable recovery. Xylazine should be given first to gain sedation. Then Telazol® is given at 1.5-2.2 mg/kg IV. 20-25 minutes of anesthesia and 30-45 minutes of recumbency is provided.
2. Butorphanol at 0.044 mg/kg can be given with the xylazine. After sedation is achieved Telazol® is given at 1.1 mg/kg giving a recumbency time of 25-35 minutes.
3. Detomidine can be given for sedation. Then Telazol® is given IV at 1.1 mg/kg. Anesthesia is about 25 minutes and recumbency about 50. Another method involves detomidine at 40 microgm/kg to provide sedation, followed by Telazol® at 1.4 mg/kg. This provides about 40 minutes of anesthesia and 70 of recumbency.

III. Maintenance of anesthesia intravenously

This method of continuing anesthesia in foals less than one month of age and very old horses is not recommended.

To reduce anesthetic related problems intravenous anesthesia should last no longer than 60-90 minutes. The veterinarian should use as little anesthetic as possible to minimize the time for recovery.

A. Thiobarbiturates (thiamylal and thiopental)

Give in increments of 0.25-0.50 gm IV to adult horses to desired effect. Maximum total dose of no more than 5.0 gm. Xylazine should be given if recovery is violent.

B. Ketamine

Additional xylazine at 0.33-0.55 mg/kg and ketamine at 0.7-1.1 mg/kg can be given to lengthen anesthesia. To gain 10-15 additional minutes of anesthesia give 1/3 of the original amounts of both drugs. Expect prolonged recovery times. Additional xylazine should be given if recovery is violent.

C. Guaifenesin and thiobarbiturate

To maintain anesthesia and to shorten recovery time reduce the amount of thiobarbiturate in each additional liter of the mixture. For example, liter #1 would have 2 gm of thiobarbiturate and liter #2 would have 1 gm, with each additional liter having 0.5-1.0 gm. (Remember, no more than 5 gm of thiobarbiturate total.)

D. Xylazine, guaifenesin and ketamine

This mixture can be used after a foal or horse has been induced with xylazine and ketamine. The mixture contains xylazine at 0.5 mg/ml, guaifenesin at 50 mg/ml and ketamine at 1-2 mg/ml. Anesthesia is maintained at 2.0-3.0 ml/kg/hr but should be adjusted as needed for each animal. If the amount of mixture expected to be used is greater than 2.2 ml/kg, then reduce the amount of ketamine in the mixture to 1.0 mg/ml OR reduce the amount of xylazine in the mixture to 0.25 mg/ml.

Calculate the rate of administration using a 15 drops/ml administration set with the following formula:

$$\frac{\text{weight of horse X dose X 15 drops/ml}}{\text{60 minutes/hr}} = \text{drops/minute}$$

The rate of infusion for a 300 kg horse would be:

$$\frac{\text{300 kg X 2 ml/kg/hr X 15 drops/ml}}{\text{60 minutes/hr}} = \text{150 drops/minute}$$

CLINICAL TECHNIQUES IN BOVINE ANESTHESIA[16]

General considerations:

1) Most of the drugs used are not approved for use in cattle. Read the label carefully and notify the owner of any extra-label use.
2) The animal's head should be positioned so that fluids from the stomach will not be aspirated during recumbency. Placing cattle in left lateral recumbency reduces the chances of regurgitation. Place padding just behind and under the

ears so that fluid will drain from the mouth rather than being aspirated.

3) Violent recoveries are not a problem as in horses so sedatives are not routinely given prior to anesthesia.

4) Cattle, except young calves, are fasted for 1-2 days and kept from water for 12-18 hours prior to an anesthetic procedure. This helps to prevent bloating and regurgitation during the recumbent period.

5) Atropine or glycopyrrolate are given if the heart rate slows below 70 beats/minute in adults or 80 in calves.

<u>I. Tranquilizers and sedatives</u>

A. Most dosages are listed in previous pages.

B. Chloral hydrate

For wild or difficult to catch cattle 30-60 gm of chloral hydrate can be added to 1-2 liters of drinking water. Onset requires 15-20 minutes and the degree of sedation varies with the animal.

C. Xylazine and butorphanol

Give xylazine at 0.01-0.02 mg/kg IV and butorphanol at 0.01-0.02 mg/kg IV at the same time but in different syringes. This combination will provide 60 minutes of standing sedation.

<u>II. Induction of anesthesia</u>

A. Thiobarbiturates (thiamylal and thiopental)

These can be given at 6.6-8.8 mg/kg rapidly IV as a 5-10% solution for adults and 2.5-5% solution for calves.

B. Guaifenesin and thiobarbiturate or guaifenesin and ketamine

50 mg guaifenesin is combined with either 2 gm thiobarbiturate or 1 gm of ketamine. The dose for unsedated cattle is 110.0 mg/kg given rapidly IV to effect. Duration of anesthesia is 15-30 minutes.

C. Xylazine, guaifenesin and ketamine

These are given together to induce and maintain anesthesia. The mixture contains 50 mg/ml of guaifenesin, 1 mg/ml ketamine, and xylazine 0.1 mg/ml. The mixture is given IV at 0.5 ml/kg.

D. Xylazine and ketamine

In calves use xylazine at 0.1-0.2 mg/kg IM, followed by ketamine at 10-15 mg/kg IM to obtain 45 minutes of anesthesia. Additional ketamine at 3-5 mg/kg can be given to lengthen anesthesia. Dose xylazine 0.03-0.05 mg/kg IV followed by ketamine at 3 mg/kg IV to obtain 20 minutes of anesthesia.

In adults give xylazine at 0.1-0.2 mg/kg IV, followed with ketamine at 2.2 mg/kg IV. Anesthesia lasts 30 minutes and can be prolonged for 15 minutes with additional ketamine at 0.75-1.25 mg/kg IV.

E. Diazepam and ketamine

Diazepam is given IV at 0.11 mg/kg in the same syringe or at the same time as ketamine at 4.4 mg/kg IV to obtain 15 minutes of anesthesia and 30 minutes of recumbency.

F. Telazol®

Telazol® can be given at 2.2-4 mg/kg IV to unsedated calves to obtain 20-60 minutes of anesthesia.

G. Xylazine and Telazol®

Xylazine given IV at 0.05 mg/kg followed by Telazol® at 1 mg/kg IV or xylazine 0.1 mg/kg IM followed immediately by Telazol® 4 mg/kg IM gives about one hour of anesthesia and up to 2 hours of recumbency.

III. Maintenance of anesthesia

A. Telazol® or ketamine or thiobarbiturates can be used to maintain anesthesia by giving 1/4 to 1/3 of the initial dose.

B. Xylazine, guaifenesin and ketamine

This combination of xylazine at 0.1 mg/ml, guaifenesin at 50 mg/ml and ketamine at 1 mg/ml can be given at 1.5 ml/kg/hr IV to calves and 2 mg/kg/hr IV to adults. The formula to calculate the volume of mixture is given in the equine anesthesia part of this section. If more than 2.2 ml/kg of the mixture is required, then the amount of xylazine should be decreased to 0.05 mg/ml so that recovery is quicker.

CLINICAL TECHNIQUES IN SHEEP AND GOAT ANESTHESIA[16]

General considerations:

Refer to those under cattle anesthesia with the following exceptions:

1) The fasting period is 12-24 hours and the period kept from water is 12 hours.

2) The heart rate is 80-150 beats/minute during anesthesia.

I. Tranquilizers and sedatives

See previous pages for drugs and doses.

II. Induction and maintenance of anesthesia

A. Thiobarbiturates (thiamylal and thiopental)

Administer these at 6.6-11.0 mg/kg IV to effect. To maintain anesthesia give additional injections (usually 1/4 to 1/3 of initial dose) to effect.

B. Guaifenesin and ketamine or guaifenesin and thiobarbiturate

The mixtures contain 50 mg/ml of guaifenesin and either 1 mg/ml of ketamine or 2.0 mg/ml of thiobarbiturate. Dose the mixture at 2.0 ml/kg and usually 50-75% of this dose is required for induction. The solution is given IV to effect using large syringes or infusion. Maintain anesthesia with either mixture given to effect.

C. Xylazine and ketamine

Goats

To produce 30-45 minutes of anesthesia give xylazine IM at 0.22 mg/kg (give atropine at 0.4 mg/kg at this time too), followed in 10 minutes by ketamine IM at 11.0 mg/kg. Maintain with 2.2-6.6 mg/kg of ketamine IM as needed. For 15-20 minutes of anesthesia give xylazine at 0.03-0.05 mg/kg IV, followed by ketamine at 3-5 mg/kg IV or alternatively give xylazine IM at 0.1 mg/kg, followed by ketamine IV at 5 mg/kg.

Sheep

To produce 30 minutes of anesthesia give xylazine at 0.22 mg/kg IM, followed in 10 minutes with ketamine at 10-15 mg/kg IM. Maintain with 2.2-6.6 mg/kg of ketamine as needed. For 15-20 minutes of anesthesia give xylazine IV at 0.03-0.05 mg/kg, followed by ketamine IV at 5 mg/kg or alternatively give xylazine IM at 0.22 mg/kg, followed by ketamine at 5 mg/kg IV.

D. Diazepam and ketamine

Goats and Sheep

Diazepam at 0.11 mg/kg IV, followed immediately by ketamine at 4.4 mg/kg IV gives 10-15 minutes of anesthesia. In sheep, diazepam at 0.25-0.5 mg/kg IV, followed immediately with ketamine at 4-7.5 mg/kg IV can also be used.

E. Acepromazine and ketamine

Sheep

Give atropine at 0.13 mg/kg IM and acepromazine at 0.55 mg/kg IV (lower doses of acepromazine should work). Ten minutes later give ketamine IV slowly at 22 mg/kg.

Maintain anesthesia by giving ketamine at 2.2-4.4 mg/kg IV.

F. Xylazine, guaifenesin and ketamine

Sheep

This combination can be used to induce and maintain anesthesia at the same concentrations as are used in cattle. The mixture is infused IV at 1.2 ml/kg for induction and 2.6 ml/kg/hr for maintenance. The formula for the calculation or the rate at which this mixture is infused can be found under equine anesthesia. Recovery is within 90 minutes of the end of infusion. If more than 2.2 ml/kg is calculated to be needed to complete the procedure, then decrease the xylazine to 0.05 mg/ml so that recovery is not delayed.

G. Telazol®

Doses above 12 mg/kg IV cause a decrease in heart and lung function, therefore an initial dose of 2.2-4.4 mg/kg IV with 1/4 to 1/3 of that dose given as needed to prolong anesthesia provides more safety, better control and a quicker recovery.

H. Telazol® and xylazine

Xylazine at 0.1 mg/kg IM, followed immediately by Telazol® at 4 mg/kg IM gives one hour of anesthesia. Recumbency lasts another hour.

I. Telazol® and butorphanol

Butorphanol at 0.5 mg/kg IV can be given 10 minutes before or at the same time as Telazol® at 4 mg/kg IV.

CLINICAL TECHNIQUES IN SWINE ANESTHESIA[16]

General considerations:

1) Intravenous access is limited. One technique uses the veins in the ears. A rubber band is placed around the base of the ear and clamped or held tightly so that the veins fill. Alcohol is used to clean and expose the veins. Enter the vein with a 20 to 22 gauge needle (or butterfly extension set or IV catheter), release the rubber band and give the injection.
2) IM injections are best given in the neck and not in the hind legs. Make sure the needle is long enough to enter the muscle since absorption of most of these drugs can be poor from fat tissue.

3) Remove food for 12 hours and water for 6 hours prior to anesthesia.
4) Atropine should be administered 15 minutes before induction at 0.044 mg/kg IM.
5) Heart rate during anesthesia should be 80-130 beats/minute

I. Tranquilizers and sedatives

A. Doses are listed in previous pages

II. Induction and maintenance of anesthesia

A. Thiobarbiturates (thiamylal and thiopental)

These can be given at 6.6-8.8 mg/kg IV as a 5% solution (50 mg/ml) through an ear vein. This amount provides 10-15 minutes of anesthesia. Maintenance can be accomplished by giving 1/4 to 1/3 of the initial dose as needed.

B. Acepromazine and ketamine

Give acepromazine at 0.4 mg/kg IM followed 30 minutes later by ketamine at 15 mg/kg IM. 60-90 minutes of restraint is obtained. Local anesthesia is often given as well to perform painful procedures.

C. Xylazine and ketamine

Give xylazine at 1.1-2.2 mg/kg IM 10 minutes before ketamine at 11-15 mg/kg IM. Anesthesia lasts 30-45 minutes. Variations in the level of anesthesia should be expected.

An alternate method involves mixing xylazine at 2.2 mg/kg and ketamine at 2.2 mg/kg and giving them IV. Anesthesia lasts 15-20 minutes.

To prolong anesthesia give 1/4 to 1/3 of the initial dose of ketamine as needed.

D. Xylazine, butorphanol and ketamine

Combine xylazine at 2.2 mg/kg, butorphanol at 0.22 mg/kg and ketamine at 11 mg/kg and give IM. Anesthesia lasts 30-45 minutes. Muscle relaxation is better than B or C. Prolong anesthesia with ketamine at 1/4 to 1/3 of initial dose.

E. Azaperone and ketamine

Give azaperone at 2.2 mg/kg IM, followed 15-45 minutes later by ketamine at 11-22 mg/kg IM. 30-45 minutes of anesthesia is provided.

Alternatively ketamine can be given IV at a reduced dose. Maintain anesthesia with additional ketamine given at 1/4 to 1/3 of the initial dose.

F. Xylazine, guaifenesin and ketamine

Mix guaifenesin at 50 mg/ml, ketamine at 1 mg/ml, and xylazine at 1 mg/ml. For induction infuse at 0.5-1.0 ml/kg IV. Maintain anesthesia at 2.0 ml/kg/hr. Recovery takes 30-60 minutes after stopping the infusion. Some animals will vomit during the recovery period.

G. Telazol® and xylazine

Telazol® should not be given IM either alone or in combination with xylazine to adult swine because of prolonged recovery time. In young swine give xylazine at 2.2 mg/kg and Telazol® at 6.0 mg/kg at the same time IM to achieve 1 hour of anesthesia.

Xylazine at 2.2 mg/kg and Telazol® at 1.0 mg/kg can be given IV at the same time or mixed in the same syringe. Xylazine can be used as the diluent for mixing Telazol® to obtain 5 mls of solution containing 100 mg/ml of each drug.

Prolong anesthesia by giving Telazol® IV at 1/4 to 1/3 of the initial dose.

H. Telazol®, xylazine and ketamine

Reconstitute Telazol® with 2.5 ml of xylazine (100 mg/ml) and 2.5 ml of ketamine (100 mg/ml). Give this at 1.0 ml/75 kg IV. Prolong anesthesia by injecting 0.5 ml/75 kg IV slowly over 1 minute.

CLINICAL TECHNIQUES IN LLAMA ANESTHESIA[17]

General considerations:

1) Adult llamas should be kept from eating for 12-18 hours and drinking for 8-12 hours prior to anesthesia. The very young llama should not be fasted or kept from water.
2) Observe the anesthetized llama for bloat and regurgitation and position to prevent such problems.
3) Pad the head of a recumbent llama to protect its prominent eyes. The down forelimb of a laterally recumbent llama should be pulled foreward to prevent damage to nerves.
4) Atropine or glycopyrrolate is not used routinely unless the heart rate drops below 30-40 beats per minute. Atropine is dosed at 0.04 mg/kg IM or 0.02 mg/kg IV.

I. Tranquilizers and sedatives

See previous pages for drugs and dosages.

II. Induction and maintenance of anesthesia

A. Xylazine and ketamine

For 30 minutes of anesthesia give xylazine at 0.4 mg/kg IM and ketamine at 4 mg/kg IM.

Alternatively, for 30-60 minutes of anesthesia give xylazine at 0.25 mg/kg IM, followed in 15 minutes by ketamine at 5 mg/kg IM.

B. Diazepam and ketamine

Mix 5-8 mg/kg of ketamine and 0.2-0.3 mg/kg of diazepam and give IM. Another method is to mix ketamine at 3-5 mg/kg and diazepam at 0.1-0.2 mg/kg and give IV.

CLINICAL TECHNIQUES IN POULTRY ANESTHESIA

General considerations:

1) Gentle handling is important in limiting stress induced heart problems
2) Subcutaneous fluids can be given in the wing webs at 15-20 ml/kg to help maintain fluid balance
3) Anesthetic depth can be tested by stimulating the wattle, comb, cere, or scaly parts of the legs with pain. These parts of the bird's body are the most sensitive, and surgery often can be performed even with these reflexes intact.
4) Body temperatures should be maintained with hot water bottles, etc.
5) Severe respiratory depression usually leads to death. Injectable anesthetics should be given carefully, usually in small doses repeated as needed rather than a single, large injection.

I. Sedation

A. Ketamine

15-20 mg/kg IM in birds weighing 500-3000 gm

B. Diazepam[20]

1-2 mg/kg IM

II. Anesthesia

A. Ketamine[20]

10-15 mg/kg IV or 15-20 mg/kg IM for birds weighing 250-2000 gm followed by incremental doses of 2-5 mg/kg to deepen to desired plane of anesthesia

B. Alfathesin[20]

10 mg/kg IV

C. Thiobarbiturates[20]

Thiamyl and thiopental at 13-26 mg/kg IV. Recovery occurs in 15-30 minutes.

D. Pentobarbitoal[20]

40-50 mg/kg in smaller birds and 15-20 mg/kg in larger ones. It has been given both IV and IM and recovery occurs in 15-30 minutes.

E. Xylazine and Ketamine

10-30 mg/kg Ketamine combined with 2-6 mg/kg xylazine in the same syringe gives 15-30 minutes of anesthesia. Best given IV although IM route also used.

ABOUT THE AUTHORS

William D. Grimley, Jr.,
Aldine Animal Hospital
440 Aldine Bender Road
Houston, TX 77060

B.S., 1980, Texas A & M University
D.V.M., 1983, Texas A & M University

Following graduation from veterinary school, Dr. Grimely practiced for a year in a mixed practice located in Hondo, Texas. Then he joined the Aldine Animal Hospital in Houston. He works primarily with dogs and cats with an occasional bird, lizard, snake, rodent, goat or horse. Dr. Grimley served on a short term mission trip to Guatemala with Christian Veterinary Mission. He and his wife Donna have three children. El está aprendiendo español para que puede llevar a cabo una obra misionera.

Randy C. Lynn,
Blue Ridge Pharmaceuticals
212 Burgess Road
Greensboro, NC 27409

B.S. 1977, The Ohio State University
M.S. 1980, The Ohio State University
D.V.M 1983, The Ohio State University
Diplomate, American College of Veterinary Clinical Pharmacology

Following graduation from veterinary school in 1983, Dr. Lynn joined the Guilford-Jamestown Veterinary Hospital as an associate before becoming owner of the Georgetown Animal Clinic in Kernersville, North Carolina in 1984. In 1985, Dr. Lynn entered corporate practice with positions at Schering Animal Health, Ciba-Geigy which became Novartis Animal Health and Blue Ridge Pharmaceuticals. He has served in Technical Services Regulatory Affairs, and in Research and Development. He now works in Research with Blue Ridge Pharmaceuticals. Dr. Lynn is a diplomate of the American College of Veterinary Clinical Pharmacology and a fellow of the American Academy of Veterinary Pharmacology and Therapeutics. He continues to work part-time in small animal practice and is active in short-term veterinary mission to Nicaragua and Honduras.

Beth Myhre Blevins,
Mixed Animal Practitioner
All Creatures Mobile Clinic
105 Rocky Bulle Road
Ronan, Montana 59864

B.A., 1982 Carrol College, Helena, MT
D.V.M., 1986, Colorado State University
Equine Internship, 1987, Washington State University

Dr. Myhre Blevins runs a solo mixed practice in Western Montana. Her 3 year old daughter Michaela is her only full-time employee while her husband Craig, who raises registered Black Angus cattle, helps her as he is able. Ethan, her son, just born in March, comes along for the ride. While working for another clinic in 1993, she hit a logging truck responding to an early morning calving call. During the 14 months recover time, she taught in a local Christian high school, had a baby, and contacted Dr. Dorminy to offer her help in writing for Christian Veterinary Mission.

Elizabeth Robinson,
2731 Paradise St.
Vernon, TX 76384

Beth Robinson received a B.S. degree in Animal Science at Louisiana State University in 1979 and graduated from the LSU School of Veterinary Medicine in 1990. Immediately after graduating, she worked in Florida for six months. She ran a relief practice in Baton Rouge for six years and has recently relocated to Vernon, TX., with her husband Don and children Erin, 13, and Clay, 9. Beth has made short-term mission trips in Haiti and on the Navajo Indian Reservation in Arizona.

We also wish to acknowledge our illustrators:
Dr. Todd Cooney, Dr. Elizabeth Robinson, Dr. Christine Appleyard.

GLOSSARY

abscess - a localized collection of pus in a cavity formed by the disintegration of tissues

absorption - the uptake of substances into or across tissues such as skin, intestine, and kidney tubules

anatomy - the science of the structure of an animal's body

anomaly - a departure from the normal. Applies particularly to those defects which are hereditary and present at birth.

antagonist - a substance that tends to cancel out the action of another substance

anthelmintic - a chemical substance which destroys worms

antibiotic - a chemical substance which inhibits the growth of or kills bacteria

antiparasitic - an agent which is destructive to parasites

antiseptic - a chemical substance which will stop or slow the growth of microorganisms. Usually used on the animal.

auscultate - to examine by listening, usually to the sounds of the thoracic or abdominal organs

aspirate - the removal of fluids or gases by the application of suction

bacteria - one-celled microorganisms which have no chlorophyll, reproduce by simple division, and can be seen only with a microscope. They occur in 3 main forms: spherical (cocci), rod-shaped (bacilli), and spiral shaped.

bolus - 1. a rounded mass of food ready to be swallowed 2. a very large tablet made to be swallowed by horses, cattle, sheep and goats 3. a concentrated mass of drug given intravenously

cancer - a growth of highly abnormal cells which spread locally and/or to other parts of the body through the blood or lymph. The natural course of this growth is often fatal.

cubic centimeter (cc) - a unit of volume in the metric system equal to a milliliter (ml)

degeneration (degenerative) - deterioration. Change of a tissue from a more organized to a less organized form.

disinfectant - a chemical which frees objects from infective microorganisms. Usually used on non-living objects.

drench - a liquid mixture of a medicine given by pouring into the back of the mouth

drug - any chemical compound that may be used or administered as an aid in the diagnosis, treatment or prevention of disease or other abnormal condition, for the relief of pain or suffering, or to control or improve any physiologic or pathologic condition

ectoparasite - a parasite that lives on the outside of the body of its host

edema - accumulation of excessive fluid in the subcutaneous tissues

endoparasite - a parasite which lives within the body of its host

esophagus - the tubular passage extending form the back of the mouth to the stomach

euthanasia - the deliberate ending of life of an animal suffering from an incurable and painful disease

exhale - to expel from the lungs by breathing

fungus - a parasitic microorganism which is found in a one cell form (yeast phase) or a multicellular form (mold) and in which no photosynthesis occurs. Fungal agents cause disease by 3 main methods: 1) invasion of living tissue by the fungus 2) allergies resulting from contact with and development of hypersensitivity to fungal antigens and 3) toxicosis resulting from eating food containing toxic metabolites of fungi.

gut sounds - sounds made by the stomach and intestines usually heard by putting one's ear or a stethoscope on the side or flank of the animal

heart girth - measurement of the distance around the body just behind the forelimbs; used in many weight estimation calculations

history - an account of information concerning an animal. It includes but is not limited to breed, sex, age, genetics, previous illnesses, previous vaccinations, housing, and food.

hydration - the relative amount of water within the body

hygiene - the science of health and of its preservation

hyperthermia - higher than normal temperature of the body

hypothermia - lower than normal temperature of the body

immune system - This system consists of a number of lymphoid organs, including the thymus, lymph nodes, spleen, parts of the liver, parts of the bone marrow, and elements in the lining of the gastrointestinal and respiratory tracts. A variety of cells that travel between the various lymphoid organs and the rest of the body make up the immune system. The immunologically active cells of the immune system compose the various classes of lymphocytes. A number of other cells, however, including monocytes, macrophages, neutrophils, eosinophils, basophils and mast cells play important accessory roles in the immune system. The role of the immune system is to defend the body against invasion by things which are foreign to it (see **immunity**).

immunity - the capacity to distinguish foreign material from self, and to neutralize, eliminate, or metabolize that which is foreign by the physiologic mechanisms of the immune response

inflammation - a localized protective response caused by injury or death of tissues. Inflammation serves to destroy, dilute, or wall off both the injurious agent and the injured tissue. It is characterized in the acute form by signs of 1. pain 2. heat 3. redness 4. swelling 5. loss of function.

inhale - to take into the lungs by breathing

intramammary - within the mammary gland or breast

intramuscular (IM) - in the muscle

intraperitoneal (IP) - in the abdominal cavity

intravenous (IV) - in the vein

ketosis - a condition characterized by an abnormally elevated concentration of ketone bodies in the body tissues and fluids. It is a complication of diabetes mellitus and starvation.

lactation - the secretion of milk

lymph system - this system consists of a network of capillaries, various sized collecting ducts, lymph nodes, and larger vessels which enter the large veins of the body. The system assists the venous portion of the blood vascular system to keep the fluids in the tissues at normal levels both in quality and quantity. The lymph nodes act as filters in the system to remove and to process infectious agents, celllular debris and other foreign material.

medicine - see **drug**

metabolism - the chemical and physical processes continuously going on in living organisms and cells. These processes include: 1) those by which ingested and absorbed food is built up into the essential matter that makes up healthy, productive cells and 2) those by which this essential matter is used and broken down into simpler substances or waste matter, with the release of energy for all vital processes in cells.

microorganism - a minute organism. Those of medical interest are bacteria, rickettsiae, viruses, molds, yeasts, and protozoa.

milligram - a unit of weight in the metric system; one one-thousandth (10^{-3} or 1/1000) of a gram

milliliter - a unit of volume in the metric system; one one-thousandth (10^{-3} or 1/1000) of a liter

mucous membrane - A membrane is a thin layer of tissue which covers a surface, lines a body cavity or divides a body space or organ. A mucous membrane is a membrane which secretes a slimy liquid made up of dead cells, salts and glandular secretions.

necropsy - examination of a body after death

ophthalmic - pertaining to the eye

oral - pertaining to the mouth

organ - a part of the body that performs a special function or functions

orthopedic - pertaining to the correction of deformities of the musculoskeletal system

otic - pertaining to the ear

palpate - to examine with the hands; to feel

pathogen - any disease producing microorganism or material

pathologic - indicative of or caused by a disease condition

pathology - that branch of medicine which studies the essential nature of disease, especially the structural and functional changes in tissues and organs of the body which cause or are caused by disease

peritoneal cavity - the abdominal cavity

physical examination - inspection of the body as a means of diagnosing disease

physiologic - characteristic of the normal functioning or state of the body, or tissue or organ

physiology - the science which studies the functions of the living organism and its parts, and of the physical and chemical factors and processes involved.

posture - the position of the body in standing or sitting

protozoa - a phylum of microscopic organisms made up of a single cell or a group of more or less identical cells and living chiefly in water, but including many parasitic forms

pulse - the rhythmic expansion of an artery which may be felt with a finger and corresponds to each beat of the heart. The pulse rate is the number of pulsations of an artery per minute.

purulent - consisting of or containing pus

pus - a liquid product of inflammation made up of cells and body fluid

respiration - the exchange of oxygen and carbon dioxide between the atmosphere and the cells of the body. The process includes inspiration and expiration, the movement of oxygen from the lungs to the blood and of carbon dioxide from the blood to the lungs, and the transport of oxygen to and carbon dioxide from the body cells.

rickettsia - a small rod-shaped to spherical microorganism which live within cells or free in the gut of lice, fleas, ticks, and mites, by which they are transmitted to man and animals

sedative - a chemical agent which decreases excitement

seizure - a violent, involuntary spasm of the muscles. A seizure can affect the entire body and is accompanied by loss of consciousness.

seroma - a collection in the tissues of serum and blood

shock - a disorder resulting from ineffective circulation of the blood, produced by blood loss, severe infection, abnormal heart function, severe trauma, etc. It is characterized by a decrease in blood pressure, rapid pulse (heart rate), and possible organ failure.

side effects - a consequence other than the one(s) for which an agent is used, especially on a tissue or organ system other than the one which it was supposed to benefit

spore (bacterial) - inactive, resistant form of a bacteria

stasis (gastrointestinal) - any condition in which normal passage of intestinal content is impaired

sterilization - the complete elimination of living microorganisms

subcutaneous (SQ or SC) - beneath the skin

symmetry - similarity of size, shape and position on either side of a dividing line or plane of the body

syndrome - a number of symptoms occurring together and characterizing a specific disease or condition

temperature - the degree of heat in a living body

tissue - a group of similarly specialized cells united in the performance of a particular function

toxicity - the quality of being poisonous

toxin - a protein which is highly poisonous for other living organisms

tranquilize - to make quiet and calm with a chemical substance (tranquilizer)

ulcer - a defect in the surface of a tissue which is produced by the sloughing of inflammatory dead tissue

virulence - the degree of pathogenicity of a microorganism as indicated by the number of deaths it has caused and/or its ability to invade the tissues of the host

virus - a group of minute infectious agents characterized by a lack of independent metabolism and by the ability to reproduce only within living host cells.

viscera - the plural form of viscus. The group of large interior organs in one of the 3 great cavities of the body, especially in the abdomen.
withdrawal period - the amount of time for removal of a medicine from the body to allow safe consumption of the meat, milk or eggs.

References

[1] Badewitz-Dodd, L.H. et al eds: *1995 IVS (Index of Veterinary Specialties) Annual, Australian Edition*, MIMS Australia, Crows Nest, NSW 1995

[2] Allen, D.G et al.: *Handbook of Veterinary Drugs*, J.B. Lippincot Co, Philadelphia, PA 1993

[3] Plumb, D.C.: *Veterinary Drug Handbook*, PharmaVet Publishing, White Bear Lake, MN 1991

[4] Brander, G.C. et. al.: *Veterinary Applied Pharmacology and Therapeutics, fifth edition*, Bailliere Tindall, Philadelphia, PA, 1991

[5] Fraser, C.M. et. al.: *The Merck Veterinary Manual, seventh edition*, Merck & Co., Rahway, NJ, 1991

[6] Johnston, D.E. ed.: *Bristol Veterinary Handbook of Antimicrobial Therapy, second edition*, Veterinary Learning Systems, 1987

[7] Howard, J.L.: *Current Veterinary Therapy; Food Animal Practice 2*, W.B. Saunders Co., Philadelphia, PA, 1986

[8] Banting, A.L. & Baggot, J.D.: *Comparison of the pharmacokinetics and local tolerance of three injectable oxytetracycline formulations in pigs*. J. Vet. Pharmacol. Ther. 19:50-55, 1996

[9] Escudero, E. et. al.: *The pharmacokinetics of a long-acting formulation of oxytetracycline in sheep and goats*. J. Vet. Pharmacol. Ther. 19:75-77, 1996

[10] Kinsell, R. & Noyer, C.L. eds: *Formulary, Purdue University School of Veterinary Medicine Pharmacy, Revised Fall 1982*. Purdue University, Lafayette, IN, 1982

[11] Morgan, R.V.: *American Animal Hospital Association, Formulary, third edition*. American Animal Hospital Association, Denver, CO, 1988.

[12] Darling, L. et. al. eds.: *Veterinary Pharmaceuticals and Biologicals, eighth edition 1993/1994.* Veterinary Medicine Publishing Co., Lenexa, KS, 1993.

[13] Lemaire, R.J. & Hosgood, G.: *Antiseptics and disinfectants in small animal practice.* Comp. Cont. Ed. Pract. Vet. 17(11):1339-1350, 1995.

[14] Marx, K.L. & Roston, M.A.: *The exotic animal drug compendium (An international Formulary)* Vet. Learning Systems, Trenton, NJ, 1996.

[15] Forney, R. & Allen, R. : *CSU Formulary* Colorado State University, Ft. Collins, Co, 1994.

[16] Riebold, T.W. , Geiser, D.R. & Goble, D.O: *Large Animal Anesthesia: Principles and Techniques,* Second Edition, Iowa State Univ. Press, 1995.

[17] Hartsfield, S.M.: *Anesthesia in Llamas.* Llama and Alpaca Symposium, Sponsored by Office of C.E., College of Vet. Med., Texas A & M Univ., February 4-5, 1995.

[18] Sander, J.E.: *Basic Information on Guinea Pigs.* Veterinary Forum, p.28, August 1992.

[19] Aeschbasher, G.: *Rabbit Anesthesia.* The Comp. Cont. Ed. Pract. Vet. 17 (8): 1004-1006, 1995.

[20] Hartsfield, S.M., McGrath, C.J.: *Anesthetic Techniques in Poultry.* Vet Clinics of N. America, Vol. 2, No. 3, Nov. 1986.

[21] United States Animal Health Association, Committee on Foreign Animal Diseases: *Foreign Animal Diseases,* fifth ed., 1992.

[22] McCurnin, D.M.: *Clinical Textbook for Veterinary Technicians,* W.B. Saunders Co., Philadelphia, PA, 1994.

[23] Patrick, C.D.: *Suggestions for Controlling External Parasites of Livestock and Poultry,* Texas Agricultural Extension Service, publication B-1306.

INDEX

Christian Veterinary Mission (Publisher of this book)

Our vision is to see

Christ's love expressed through veterinary medicine.

Our mission is to

challenge, empower and facilitate veterinarians to serve through their profession, living out their Christian faith.

CVM also provides education and encouragement for those who desire to minister through service, prayer, relationship building, and modeling Christ's love.

About CVM

Christian Veterinary Mission (CVM) is a registered non-profit Christian Service Organization 501(c)(3) based in Seattle, Washington, U.S.A.

CVM was founded in 1976 by Dr. Leroy Dorminy who came to realize the impact that veterinarians could have by integrating their faith with their practice, both locally and around the world. In 2008, CVM had nearly 30 veterinary professionals serving full-time internationally and over 200 veterinary professionals and student volunteers serve on short-term cross-cultural mission trips annually. CVM sponsors fellowship & prayer breakfasts at over 20 U.S. veterinary meetings each year and reaches out to veterinary students through Christian Veterinary Fellowship (CVF) groups in every veterinary school in the U.S. by encouraging them in spiritual growth and professional development.

There are over 3,500 veterinarians affiliated with CVM in the U.S. CVM also partners with organizations and networks in other countries that are focused on empowering Christian veterinarians. CVM has a volunteer advisory board of veterinarians who guide its vision, mission, and programming.

CVM books and the free International Animal Health Newsletter were written with small farmers, veterinarians, and agricultural development workers in mind. Our desire is that they would help individuals and groups develop an appropriate livestock program to meet community needs. CVM's Endowment Fund was started in the early years of the organization's life. The fund provides for meaningful programs that could not be funded by the regular budgeting process.

Made in the USA
Monee, IL
22 April 2022

95228965R00149